Complications in the Management of Breast Disease

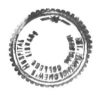

Complications in Surgery Series
Edited by John A. R. Smith

Other volumes in this series

Forthcoming volumes

Complications in the Management of Breast Disease

edited by

R. W. Blamey

Professor of Surgical Science, City Hospital, Nottingham

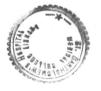

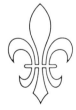

Baillière Tindall London Philadelphia Toronto
Mexico City Rio de Janeiro Sydney Tokyo Hong Kong

M 9003
20/11/86

Baillière Tindall   1 St Anne's Road
W. B. Saunders   Eastbourne, East Sussex BN21 3UN, England

West Washington Square
Philadelphia, PA 19105, USA

1 Goldthorne Avenue
Toronto, Ontario M8Z 5T9, Canada

Apartado 26370—Cedro 512
Mexico 4, DF Mexico

Rua Evaristo da Veiga 55, 20° andar
Rio de Janeiro—RJ, Brazil

ABP Australia Ltd, 44–50 Waterloo Road
North Ryde, NSW 2113, Australia

Ichibancho Central Building, 22-1 Ichibancho
Chiyoda-ku, Tokyo 102, Japan

10/fl, Inter-Continental Plaza, 94 Granville Road
Tsim Sha Tsui East, Kowloon, Hong Kong

First published 1986

Printed in Great Britain at the Alden Press, Oxford

British Library Cataloguing in Publication Data

Complications in the management of breast disease.
    —(Complications in surgery series)
    1. Breast—Cancer—Surgery
    2. Breast—Surgery—Complications and surgery
    I. Blamey, R.W.   II. Series
    616.99′449   RD667.5

ISBN 0-7020-1131-2

Contents

Series Foreword

All doctors who are involved in the care of surgical patients are all too aware of the hazards of the operation and the morbidity and mortality that can result from an ill considered or ill managed procedure, and of the complications, whether related directly to the operation, the disease process, the patient or even to the hospital environment. It is also true to say that many hospitals are now mindful of these difficulties and have introduced a pattern of regular medical audit through which the extent and the significance of the problem can be identified and which, when necessary, can point to the remedy.

The majority of complications are of course preventable by careful preoperative preparation, by skilled operative technique and by proper postoperative care, but when they do occur, it is the early recognition, the immediate and correct investigation, and the awareness of the operative treatment that will decide the eventual outcome and the likelihood of early recovery.

Obviously every surgeon would like to believe that in his own practice complications will be, at the least, occasional events and hopefully this is the case in most hospitals. The corollary of this is, however, that the personal experience of many surgeons in these serious potential or actual problems is not great and the opportunities for the trainee surgeon to learn about them, and about their clinical significance and management, are less than adequate.

This deficiency of experience in the average surgeon, whether general surgeon or specialist, has now been appreciated and John Smith in this series of texts has set out to provide what has been termed a 'reference point' from which the surgeon will be able to increase his awareness of the problems and increase his knowledge in areas where he is unlikely to gain experience from clinical practice. The prime aim of the series has been to ensure that knowledge of the existence of complications increases, that prevention can become more widely accepted and that the recognition and management of established complications can be undertaken with skill and competence.

Each of the volumes in the series considers a specific area of surgical practice and, in each, authorities in the field have presented their experience and their views in such a way that it will not only instruct but will also stimulate the reader to study the subject further.

It is undoubtedly an area of surgical practice that is of major importance and which has been somewhat neglected in the past. This is the first time that there has been an attempt to present a comprehensive account covering all aspects of practice and it

will undoubtedly be a significant contribution to patient care in
its broadest interpretation.

Sir James Fraser Bt, PPRCS (Ed)
Nicolson Street
Edinburgh

Editor's Foreword

Most textbooks of surgery acknowledge that postoperative complications exist and some describe methods of prevention or options for their further management. However, it is clear to me from conversations with junior staff, candidates for higher degrees and trainees in all branches of surgery that there is no reference to which they can turn where the complex problem of complications is adequately considered, i.e. covering details of aetiology, predisposition and methods of prevention, together with advice on which complications are likely to be encountered and how they may be recognized, investigated and managed.

This series is directed at all surgical trainees and also at the consultant working outside specialist referral centres. The latter may not often encounter the complications which are under consideration, but when they are encountered the surgeon needs advice on what to do, what not to do and, finally, when specialist referral is indicated.

The authors in this series are all consultants with a specialist practice in teaching hospitals. Each has been asked to provide the necessary information and to be dogmatic where that is possible, but to advise on the options where the situation is less clear.

Each volume is self-sufficient, except that *Complications of Surgery in General* deals with all general surgical complications to avoid detailed repetition in the other, more specialist, volumes. Inevitably there is some overlap between volumes but I feel this to be preferable to omitting topics that may be important. This is the only truly multi-author contribution to the series, resulting from the specialist nature of the complications described.

Finally, not all the complications described have been created by the authors; the selection of topic reflects, rather, their ability to deal with such problems as are referred to them!

The concept of a single volume on *Complications in Surgery* arose from discussions involving, on separate occasions, Mrs Ann Saadi (lately of Baillière Tindall), Mr R. M. Kirk (Royal Free Hospital, London) and myself. The volume has grown into a series but acknowledgements are due to Mrs Saadi and Mr Kirk for the idea and to Mrs Saadi for the enthusiasm which ensured the launch. I am most grateful to Dr Geoffrey Smaldon, lately of Baillière Tindall, who assumed responsibility for the entire series and encouraged or cajoled as necessary. Finally, I am happy to acknowledge the support and encouragement of my wife and family.

John A. R. Smith
Northern General Hospital
Sheffield

Preface

My initial reaction to being asked to write *'Complications in Surgery—Breast Disease'* was that wound infection was the sole complication of breast surgery. Breast disease does present many difficult problems of *management*. The intention of this book is (i) to identify and discuss specific problems which arise in the management of breast cancer, (ii) to discuss the complications of the treatment of breast cancer, and (iii) to identify problems of benign breast disease. In each section current objectives, results and benefits are stated but the emphasis is on the difficulties that present and on complications that arise.

The book assumes that the bases of breast disease are familiar to the reader. It is aimed at the clinician (consultant) who may be faced with these very problems in individual cases, at clinicians (consultant or research fellow) who are about to study a particular aspect of breast disease and are looking for a starting base for their study, and at trainees in a number of fields (surgery, radiology, oncology, pathology, radiotherapy) who have a general interest in the field of breast disease. Primarily I hope that the book will be used as a reference manual by clinicians who are trying to cope with a particular problem in the management of breast disease.

Although this volume of *Complications in Surgery* is multi-authored, the majority of the authors work or have worked in the Nottingham/Tenovus Breast Project based at Nottingham City Hospital. I have also exercised considerable editorial powers to try to present the book as a view from a single unit and the management plan is based on the considerable experience of the Nottingham City Hospital breast clinics. These clinics encompass patients referred to a single surgeon (RWB) with long-term follow-up. There are in addition two early detection clinics. All histopathological aspects of these cases are studied under the direction of Dr Christopher Elston. One radiotherapist (Dr David Morgan), two radiologists specializing in mammography (Dr Eric Roebuck and Dr Adrian Manhire) and one bone radiologist (Dr Alan Morris) are responsible for care and investigations within their fields. We have for the past 11 years seen around 2000 new patients per year and treated over 150 new breast cancers per year. Steroid receptor assays are carried out at the Tenovus Institute, Cardiff, under the direction of Professor Keith Griffiths and Dr Robert Nicholson. In ten instances I thought our experience of the particular problem insufficient and have asked authors with a particular interest in these situations to contribute chapters.

I am extremely grateful to my co-authors for their excellent contributions and for allowing me the exercise of editorial red pen. I would particularly like to thank our guest contributors for joining the Nottingham authors. I wish to thank Tenovus for their years of help with breast cancer management and research in Nottingham.

Roger Blamey

List of Contributors

Contributors from Nottingham City Hospital and Tenovus Institute

Roger Blamey, Professor of Surgical Science

Christopher Elston, Consultant Histopathologist

David Morgan, Consultant Radiotherapist

Eric Roebuck, Consultant Radiologist

Charles Campbell, Tenovus Research Fellow in Surgery (1981–83)

Howard Holliday, Research Fellow in Surgery (1979–81)

Christopher Hinton, Research Fellow in Surgery (1982–84)

Michael Williams, Tenovus Research Fellow in Surgery

Peter Blacklay, Surgical Registrar (1981)

Iain Muir, Surgical Registrar (1984)

Clive Griffith, Lecturer in Surgery

Richard Blake, Lecturer in Surgery (1978–84)

Susan Mann, Anaesthetist

Robert Nicholson, Scientific Officer, Tenovus Institute for Cancer Research, Cardiff

Guest contributors

Richard Bennett is Professor of Surgery, University of Melbourne (St Vincent's Hospital)

Charles Galasko is Professor of Orthopaedic Surgery, Manchester University, Hope Hospital

Penelope Hopwood is Research Senior Registrar, University Hospital of South Manchester

Adrian L. Harris is Professor of Clinical Oncology, The University of Newcastle-upon-Tyne

Jillian Haslehurst is Medical Officer, Marks & Spencer Ltd

Michael Kettlewell is Consultant Surgeon, The John Radcliffe Hospital, Oxford

Patricia Clarke is Surgical Registrar, Oxford

Peter Maguire is Senior Lecturer in Psychiatry, University Hospital of South Manchester

John Miles is Consultant Neurosurgeon, Associated Unit of Neurological Science, The University of Liverpool

Paul Preece is Senior Lecturer in Surgery, University of Dundee

John Simpson is Senior Lecturer in Surgery, University of Wellington, New Zealand

1 The Diagnosis of Breast Cancer

Christopher Elston and Roger Blamey

The commonest way in which a breast cancer first presents is as a palpable lump in the breast. The other presentations—mammographic abnormality, soreness of the nipple, discharge from the nipple, and metastases in distant sites or in axillary nodes—are much less common. Mammographic abnormalities leading to the diagnosis of cancer are increasing as screening programmes are introduced. Soreness of the nipple due to underlying Paget's disease accounts for only 1% of the breast cancers in the Nottingham–Tenovus series. Discharge from the nipple has led to only five cancers being diagnosed (out of approximately 2500); distant metastasis with a previously unrecognized small palpable primary has been seen only three times as the presenting sign. Metastasis to axillary nodes without palpable lump has accounted for seven presentations.

Breast lump
Unfortunately, in the enthusiasm for newer means of diagnosis, patients complaining of breast lumps are often improperly managed. In the Nottingham Breast Clinic the first decision that the clinician must make is whether a lump is present or not. The decision that a lump is present must be clear and means that the patient is committed to surgery unless the lump proves cystic on needling. In some cases the surgeon is sure that there is no lump; this is an easier decision in the postmenopausal or the teenage breast. In other cases the surgeon feels no definite lump but the breast is generally lumpy and this is frequently so in the women of 35 to 50 years of age. These patients are seen again six weeks later, at a different phase of their menstrual cycle; if the breast is unduly lumpy on that occasion, then the patient is sent for mammography. This raises a further point: if the examiner decides that a lump is present then mammography is not employed at this stage since it contributes nothing further to diagnosis.

These points have been stressed because we feel strongly that they are important principles. Clear thinking and definite decisions must be made and there must be no abdication from clinical decision by substitution of mammography.

Once the decision is made that a lump is present, then the surgeon proceeds on a set path. A 21-gauge needle is advanced

Figure 1.1
Core obtained by
Trucut needle.

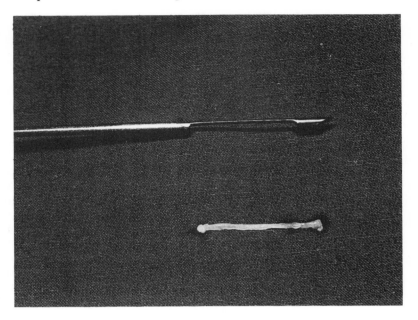

into the lump and an attempt made to aspirate fluid; if a lump proves to be a cyst and disappears completely on aspiration, then no further action is taken at this time. If the lump is solid the surgeon proceeds to a tissue biopsy employing either a Trucut needle for histology or fine-needle aspiration for cytology.

Trucut needle biopsy

Trucut biopsy is carried out under local anaesthetic (Elston et al, 1978). A small incision is made through the skin with the tip of a sharp scalpel blade, the Trucut needle is pushed through the skin incision, and a biopsy of the lump is taken (Fig. 1.1). Following biopsy the patient is instructed to apply firm pressure for 10 minutes: this prevents bruising. Fortunately, a carcinoma is easier to biopsy than a benign lump. The carcinoma is hard and is cut easily, while benign tissue has the consistency of firm India rubber—fibroadenomas are often too firm to push the needle into at all.

Over an eleven year period over 2000 biopsies have been taken in the referral clinic in Nottingham.

In the cases that ultimately proved to be a carcinoma, Trucut biopsy showed unequivocal cancer in 76% (Table 1.1). A further 5% of biopsies were considered 'suspicious but not diagnostic of cancer'. All such reports have proved subsequently to be from cancer cases.

It has proved possible to make diagnoses other than cancer: fibroadenoma and phyllodes tumour have been correctly diagnosed. These lumps have subsequently been removed.

With the exception of abscess and pregnant tissue (see Chapter 3), a report of benign tissue, or a report of an unsatisfactory core

Table 1.1
Trucut biopsy results from 932 cases subsequently diagnosed to be breast cancer.

Trucut diagnosis	No.	%
Carcinoma	704	76
Suspicious	44	5
Benign	180	19
	932	100

for examination, is followed by excision of the lump. Only if there is a strong clinical suspicion of cancer is frozen-section examination of the lump used. A report 'suspicious but not diagnostic of cancer' is likewise usually followed by frozen section after discussion with the patient. A report of invasive carcinoma is followed without further diagnostic procedure by the appropriate treatment. Depending on the line of treatment to be followed, a report of carcinoma without invasive change may be followed by excision of the lump to confirm or deny its in situ nature, before proceeding to definitive treatment.

There has been one false positive diagnosis of carcinoma, amounting to 0.05% of all the carcinomas, in a patient subsequently shown to have a fibroadenoma. This is approximately the rate found with frozen-section examination of a lump.

Fine-needle aspiration cytology (Fig. 1.2)

A preoperative diagnosis can also be achieved using fine-needle aspiration cytology. In the most frequently used method a 21-gauge 40 mm needle is attached to a 10 ml syringe and the needle is passed into the lump in several directions whilst applying suction. Smears are air dried and stained by the May–Grunwald–Giemsa method.

Figure 1.2
Carcinoma cells obtained at fine needle aspiration cytology. May–Grunwald Giemsa ×730.

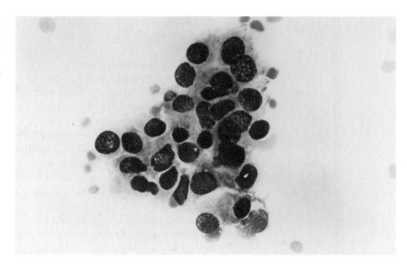

Figure 1.3
Benign epithelial cells
from a fibroadenoma
obtained at fine
needle aspiration
cytology. May–Grun-
wald Giemsa ×730.

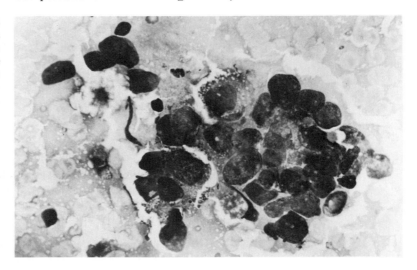

In most studies accurate diagnosis of carcinoma is achieved in over 90% of cases, when technically inadequate samples are excluded. These may amount to 25% of cases (Furnival et al, 1975) and the only way to reduce this to a satisfactory level is to examine the smears immediately and repeat the aspiration if necessary. This is a disadvantage of the method as it requires the cytologist to be available for the whole of a clinic. False positive diagnoses do occur, and the lesions are nearly always shown subsequently to be fibroadenomas (Fig. 1.3). In view of this, some centres always confirm a cytological diagnosis in young women by frozen-section biopsy.

It must be stressed that to achieve a high standard of diagnostic accuracy special training in breast cytology is mandatory. This is not a method that should be practised by pathologists undertaking routine cervical cytology without such training (Elston et al, 1978).

Diagnosis from mammography

Mammography is not a diagnostic method for use in the referral clinic. Mammography may occasionally prove a useful adjunct, but should never be used to replace clear clinical decisions.

The present use of mammography in the referral clinic is restricted to the investigation of cases where the breasts are too 'lumpy' to discount the possibility that a discrete lump is present. We try to keep this group to a minimum. Thus, cases are put into three categories: definite lump (investigated as above), definitely 'no lump' (usually these cases are seen a second time six weeks later at the opposite phase of their menstrual cycle), and too lumpy to be certain that no lump is present (these cases are sent for mammography and seen again six weeks later).

Mammography is, however, the basis of breast screening

Figure 1.4
Marker biopsy of
impalpable lesion
seen on mammogram.
This lesion closely
mimics a carcinoma
but is, in fact, a radial
scar (see Chapter 3).

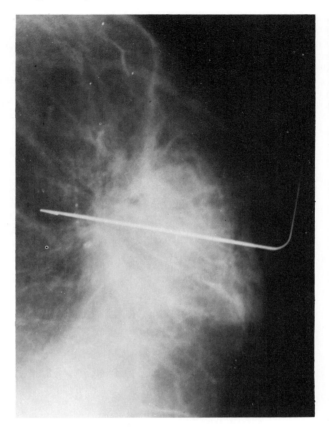

programmes (Chapter 7). It is a very efficient method of detecting impalpable carcinomas. Such lesions shown only on mammography are removed by 'marker-biopsy' in which the radiologist places a fish-hooked needle in the position in which the abnormality has been detected (Fig. 1.4) under mammographic control. This needle must be taped carefully to the skin in order to avoid the needle migrating into the breast or, worse, into the pleural cavity. The patient is taken to theatre and the tissue around the needle point is excised under general anaesthetic. The tissue is then sent for X-ray to confirm that the mammographic lesion is contained within the biopsy.

In order to keep the ratio of benign to malignant biopsies to a reasonable level, the radiologist should grade his reporting and not simply report the presence of any abnormality (see Chapter 8).

Paget's disease of the nipple
Paget's disease of the nipple (Fig. 1.5) should be suspected in any patient presenting with rawness of the nipple—a rawness some-

Figure 1.5
Paget's disease of the nipple. Groups of large carcinoma cells are seen infiltrating amongst the smaller darker staining keratinocytes. H&E ×490.

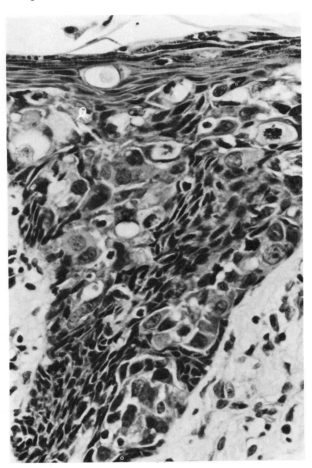

times restricted to the nipple and sometimes extending to the areola. Some of these cases have a palpable lump, which is investigated as above. The remainder are investigated by nipple biopsy. This is a simple process, performed in the referral clinic with a sharp scalpel blade under local anaesthetic containing a little adrenaline to diminish skin bleeding, and with insertion of one stitch.

Cases confirmed as Paget's disease are then investigated mammographically. The managment of Paget's disease where it is confined to the nipple, with no underlying palpable or mammographic lesion, is debatable. Until recently we used a cone biopsy of the nipple only. However there were several local recurrences of the disease and at present we suggest that even lesions as localized as this should undergo mastectomy.

Nipple discharge
Few carcinomas present as nipple discharge alone, although it is

a symptom often stressed in women's magazines and indeed in lectures to medical students. In fact, in the Nottingham clinic only five carcinomas have been discovered from investigation of nipple discharge alone. Our management of nipple discharge is described in Chapter 4.

Breast cancer presenting as metastases

Over 2000 breast cancers have come under our care in the last ten years. Seven have presented as enlarged axillary nodes showing adenocarcinoma on histological examination when no lump was palpable nor mammographic lesion initially visible; two cases were placed under observation and cancers presented ultimately in the ipsilateral breast; in one case mastectomy was carried out but careful examination of the breast failed to reveal a carcinoma; the others revealed breast cancer at mastectomy.

Two cases were diagnosed after presenting initially as bony metastases. In both, a small but palpable primary breast cancer was present.

Controversies and Future Developments
- The regular use of fine needle cytology—requires a pathologist with particular expertise in each centre.
- Better mammographic reading—requires a radiologist with expertise.
- As a consequence of the above, more specialist breast clinics.
- Referral for mammography in the symptomatic case only after a specialist clinical examination.

References

Elston, C.W., Cotton, R.E., Davies, C.J. & Blamey, R.W. (1978) A comparison of the use of the 'Tru-cut' needle and fine needle aspiration cytology in the preoperative diagnosis of carcinoma of the breast. *Histopathology*, 2, 239–254.

Furnival, C.M., Hocking, M.A., Hughes, H.E. et al (1975) Aspiration cytology in breast cancer: its relevance to diagnosis. *Lancet*, ii, 446–449.

2 Borderline Lesions

Christopher Elston and Roger Blamey

The term 'borderline lesion' is used increasingly in breast disease, although in practice it is difficult to produce a definition which is entirely satisfactory. For the purposes of this chapter we have made an arbitrary decision to consider (1) 'benign' epithelial proliferations which appear to have premalignant potential and (2) in situ carcinoma. These cover the spectrum of lesions which lie between those which are definitely benign and those which show invasive malignancy. Such lesions have assumed much greater importance in recent years owing to the increasing use of mammography and the introduction of screening programmes. This has placed an additional burden on the histopathologist whose opinion in this difficult area determines the treatment policy.

Epithelial proliferation with premalignant potential

Mammary dysplasia is the commonest non-malignant breast lesion in premenopausal women. It usually presents as a palpable lump, or as 'lumpy' breasts, because of the cystic component or associated stromal fibrosis. The histological changes occur in the terminal duct–lobular unit owing to abnormalities in cyclical proliferation and regression of both epithelial and stromal elements. The characteristic features are cyst formation, interlobular fibrosis, duct ectasia, apocrine metaplasia and a variable degree of epithelial proliferation. Since Warren in 1940 suggested that benign mammary dysplasia increased the risk of subsequent breast cancer by four times, the subject has been surrounded by considerable controversy. Despite numerous studies which have supported this concept there has not been universal acceptance. Many studies have been based on inadequate numbers of patients, or have been retrospective, in some histology was not reviewed, and ill-defined terminology has hampered comparisons between different centres. It should further be noted that the assessment of histological changes can be based on biopsy material submitted on the basis of the clinical judgement exercised by a surgeon. No assumption can be made from such biopsies concerning changes in the rest of the breast, and it must also be appreciated that similar changes are almost certainly present in the breasts of age-matched women who do not present for clinical examination. Nevertheless, in studies which have considered the individual components which make up mammary dysplasia, more convincing evidence has been presented to suggest that women with epithelial proliferation do have an

Figure 2.1
Epitheliosis in mammary dysplasia, with a duct in the centre filled with epithelial cells. H&E ×120.

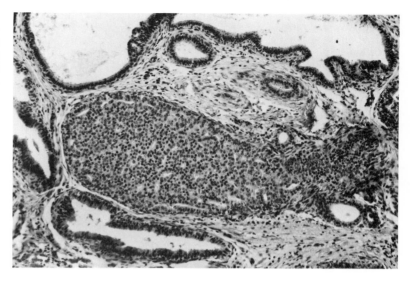

increased risk of breast cancer (Black et al, 1972; Page et al, 1978; Dupont and Page, 1985). Epithelial proliferation can be considered in two main groups:

Ductal   In the United Kingdom and Europe, the term epitheliosis (Figs 2.1 and 2.2) is used to denote the benign proliferation of epithelial cells which occur mainly in the subsegmental and terminal ducts. The same lesion is referred to as papillomatosis in the United States. This is unfortunate since the changes seen are not necessarily papillary and confusion with genuine duct papillo-

Figure 2.2
Higher power view of duct shown in Figure 2.1. The cells are regular in size and shape. H&E ×450.

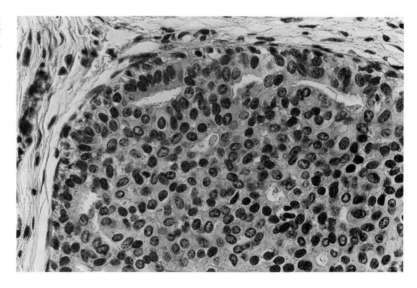

Figure 2.3
Atypical ductal
hyperplasia. There
is a disorderly pro-
liferation of epithelial
cells with irregular
'bridging'. Slight var-
iation in nucleus size
is seen. H&E ×315.

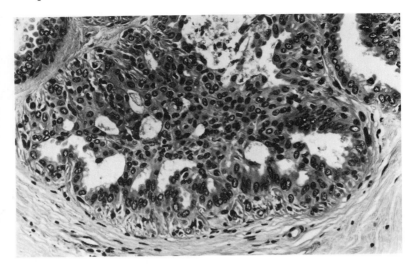

mas may be caused. Page and co-workers (Page et al, 1985; Dupont and Page, 1985) use the term ductal hyperplasia, which is more acceptable. The number of ducts involved is very variable, and in some cases the change is florid. The lumen of the ducts is filled with large epithelial cells which usually have abundant cytoplasm. There is often a 'streaming' type of growth pattern, and small capillaries and myoepithelial cells may be distinguished within the proliferating cells. Nuclei tend to be regular in appearance without significant atypia. Mitoses are infrequent and normal in configuration. Cell necrosis is not seen.

Figure 2.4
Atypical lobular
hyperplasia. The
acini contain a pro-
liferation of epithelial
cells, but lumina are
present and there is
no increase in acinar
size. H&E ×450.

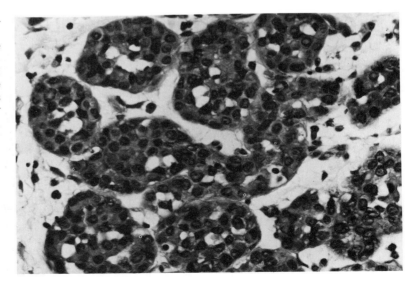

Figure 2.5
Intraduct carcinoma.
There is epithelial
proliferation with
marked variation in
nuclear size and
shape. H&E ×450.

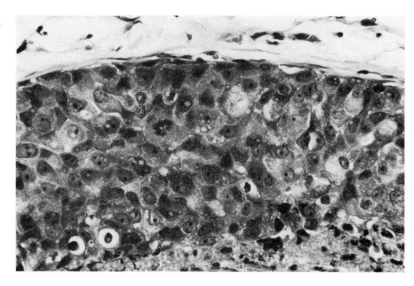

In the uncommon variant termed atypical ductal hyperplasia (Page et al, 1978) epithelial 'bridging' and cytological atypia are suggestive of in-situ carcinoma, but the overall appearances do not warrant a diagnosis of malignancy (Fig. 2.3).

Lobular   The term atypical lobular hyperplasia is applied to the proliferation of epithelial cells within a lobule or group of lobules (Fig. 2.4) which does not fulfil the criteria accepted for lobular carcinoma-in-situ. The epithelial cells are small and regular with central nuclei and scanty cytoplasm. The lobules are not usually

Figure 2.6
Solid type of intra-
duct carcinoma
showing obliteration
of the lumen by proli-
ferating atypical cells.
H&E ×180.

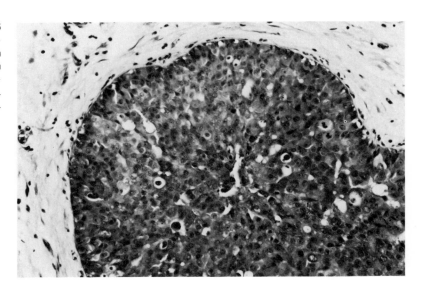

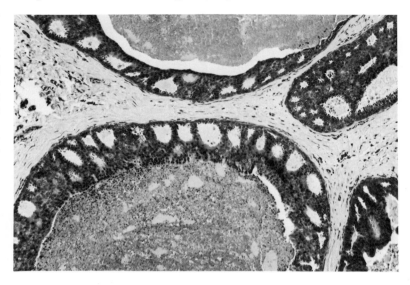

Figure 2.7 Cribriform type of intraduct carcinoma. Note the lacy network of epithelial cells at the periphery of ducts with a 'Roman bridge' effect. Note the central necrotic 'comedo' debris. H&E ×120.

expanded in size, acinar distension is minimal, and lumina persist. The number of lobules involved is variable, and only partial involvement of individual lobules may be seen. Nuclear atypia is rare and mitoses are infrequent.

In-situ malignancy

By conventional definition an in-situ carcinoma is one in which there is cytological evidence of malignancy in the epithelial cells of the organ or structure in question, but in which the basement

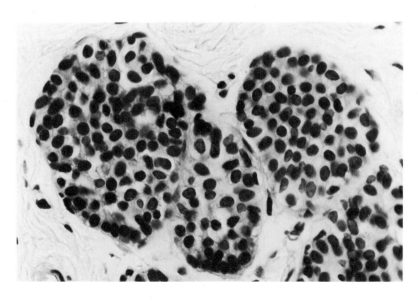

Figure 2.8 Lobular carcinoma-in-situ. Acini are expanded by a solid proliferation of epithelial cells, obliterating the lumina. H&E ×670.

membrane remains intact and there is no evidence of stromal invasion. In-situ carcinoma of the breast is subdivided into two types, based on the presumed site of origin within the terminal duct–lobular unit:

Intraduct carcinoma

A variable number of ducts is involved, and the lesion may be confined to one quadrant of the breast or be multifocal. Ducts are usually dilated, with intact, often thickened, basement membranes and periductal fibrosis and inflammation may be conspicuous features. Large epithelial cells with abundant cytoplasm proliferate in a disorderly fashion within the ducts. The cells vary in size and shape and there is nuclear atypicality with an increased mitotic activity (Fig. 2.5). Three main microscopical patterns are recognized although these appear to have no prognostic significance. In the *solid* type the ducts are filled with tumour cells which become closely packed and may appear polyhedral; the lumen is obliterated (Fig. 2.6). The cribriform variant is characterized by the formation of apparent glandular spaces within the proliferating tumour cells, giving a lacy network appearance (Fig. 2.7). The *comedo* type is so termed because the tumour cells in the centre of the duct lumen breaks down to form an amorphous lipid-rich secretion which can be expressed on pressure like an acne comedo. Frequently only a few layers of cells survive around the periphery of involved ducts. All three types may be present in the same tumour or there may be combination of any two (Fig. 2.7).

Lobular carcinoma-in-situ

Like intraduct carcinoma, this lesion may be confined to one area of the breast or be multifocal. Thus a variable number of lobules is involved by a proliferation of small darkly-staining epithelial cells. The lobules are usually enlarged and each acinus is filled and distended with obliteration of the lumen (Fig. 2.8). As a result of the enlargement of acini, the intralobular connective-tissue stroma appears relatively reduced. Nuclei are regular, and atypical cells and mitoses are infrequent. Proliferating cells may extend into the terminal duct in a 'Pagetoid' fashion.

Although both intraduct carcinoma and lobular carcinoma-in-situ are by definition in-situ lesions, multiple blocks must be examined in each case to exclude the possibility of early invasion.

Discussion

In assessing the importance of borderline lesions of the breast in clinical practice, it is important to appreciate their comparative rarity. Breast lesions showing epithelial proliferation account for less than a third and those with cellular atypia less than 2% of benign breast biopsies in our series. In-situ carcinoma constitutes approximately 3% of all malignant lesions. This is in accord with published data: Dupont and Page (1985) found that only 26% of consecutive benign breast biopsies showed proliferative changes, and 4% had cellular atypia, while in the United Kingdom Trial of Early Detection of Breast Cancer the categories of epithelial proliferation with atypia and in-situ carcinoma account for 2.5% of all biopsies. In routine practice, therefore, these lesions will be encountered relatively infrequently, and in a small minority of patients.

Histopathologically, the diagnosis of proliferative epithelial lesions in the breast may be extremely difficult. To a large extent this is due to the clinical requirement for the pathologist to assign a lesion definitely to the benign or malignant category, while in reality there is a spectrum of changes with no rigid dividing line. In practice, the important cut-off point lies between epithelial proliferation with atypia and in-situ carcinoma.

The criteria for in-situ carcinoma proposed by McDivitt et al (1968) and Azzopardi (1979) are now generally accepted and should form the basis for the diagnosis of difficult lesions. Not surprisingly there is less agreement concerning the hyperplastic epithelial proliferations. Most of the difficulty is caused by terminological differences. The designation of epitheliosis in the United Kingdom and papillomatosis in the United States for the same lesion has already been discussed. The concept that a small group of atypical ductal hyperplasias can be identified, is now gaining support (Page et al, 1985). The assessment of lobular epithelial proliferations produces the greatest difficulty in diagnosis. In the first formal report of lobular carcinoma-in-situ by Foote and Stewart, cases were included which would now undoubtedly be regarded as benign. Foote and Stewart advocated that all patients with these lesions should be treated by mastectomy, and this view was widely accepted, especially in the United States. Haagensen et al (1978) recognized that this was too draconian an approach and proposed that non-infiltrative lobular proliferations be termed lobular neoplasia and treated conservatively by local excision with regular follow-up. This terminology has not found universal acceptance, and most authorities now recommend the use of the term atypical lobular hyperplasia if a lobular proliferation does not have all the features required for lobular carcinoma-in-situ to be diagnosed (Page et al, 1985). It is certainly easier to persuade surgeons to manage a patient conservatively if a benign rather than a malignant name has been applied to a lesion, but this places considerable pressure on the pathologist to ensure that his diagnostic criteria are correct.

Because of the conflicting evidence regarding the relative risk for subsequent invasive carcinoma in women with benign breast disease, there has been little agreement about the appropriate management for these patients. Recent studies would now seem to have resolved many of the uncertainties, and more definite management protocols can be envisaged. Dupont and Page (1985), have now shown that risk is only related to specific proliferative abnormalities. Thus women whose biopsies do not show epithelial proliferation have no increased risk. Since this category accounts for 70% of all non-malignant biopsies, the great majority of women can be reassured and do not require follow-up. The presence of epithelial proliferation increases the lifetime risk of breast cancer twofold, and such biopsies account for 5% of biopsies. Epithelial atypia gives the most significant association, with an increased risk of just over four times. This risk is doubled if the patient has a family history of breast cancer. However, atypia was only found by Dupont and Page in 4% of biopsies, and atypia with family history in less than 1% of patients. Long-term follow-up can certainly be justified in the very small group of patients with atypia, especially if there is a family history, but there appears to be no benefit from conducting follow-up in patients with proliferative lesions without atypia. To put the problem into perspective, it is worth noting that only one patient in 50 with breast cancer has had previous breast surgery (Chetty et al, 1980).

The management of patients with in-situ carcinoma has been equally contentious. The apparent logic is that the less dangerous the lesion the greater the chance of success of therapy with breast conservation. However, the great majority of those patients with diagnosed in-situ carcinoma are going to live for a long time and not present with distant metastases (those that do so have presumably foci of invasive carcinoma which were undetected at the time of original diagnosis). In addition, a good number of in-situ carcinomas are multifocal, especially if lobular in type. We have only a small series of in-situ carcinomas treated by excision followed by irradiation (Chapter 12), but our experience in this series is sufficiently frightening to warrant report: of the seven patients, three have recurrences at the site of the tumour excision and two of these show invasive cancer on recurrence. Harris et al (1983) have reported from Boston that one of the features correlating with recurrence in the breast is the presence of in-situ carcinoma around the lesion. It is possible that in-situ carcinoma is not sensitive to irradiation to the same degree as invasive carcinoma.

With these points in mind—the length of time the patient has to live following treatment, multifocality, possible insensitivity to irradiation and the fact of invasive recurrences replacing an original curable lesion—we at present recommend for carcinoma-in-situ excision of the whole breast tissue, whether by simple mastectomy or subcutaneous mastectomy (Chapter 11).

This leaves the problem of the opposite breast. There is a great deal of argument regarding the absolute incidence of subsequent cancer of the opposite breast, but the clear fact is that the chance of this occurring is higher than the risk (for both breasts) of the women without previous breast cancer. In addition, the risk is higher in the case of lobular carcinoma in-situ. Chaudary et al (1984) report that in women with invasive cancer the incidence of subsequent cancer of the opposite breast is constant annually over the 20 years following the first carcinoma. A reasonable guess of the cumulative effect is that one woman in four will contract cancer of the opposite breast over 20–30 years. Thus authors have advocated bilateral mastectomy at the diagnosis of the first in-situ cancer especially for lobular carcinoma-in-situ. Others have suggested 'mirror-image' biopsy of the opposite breast. Our own preference is for regular (six monthly) clinical examination, the teaching of self-examination of the breast, and biennial mammography.

References

Azzopardi, J. (1979) *Problems in Breast Pathology.* London: W.B. Saunders.

Black, M.M., Barclay, T.H.C., Cutler, S.J. et al (1972) Association of atypical characteristics of benign breast lesions with subsequent risk of breast cancer. *Cancer, 29,* 338–343.

Chaudary, M.A., Millis, R.R., Hoskins, E.O.L. et al (1984) Bilateral primary breast cancer: a prospective study of disease incidence. *Br. J. Surg., 71,* 711–714.

Chetty, U., Wang, C.C., Forrest, A.P.M. & Roberts, M.M. (1980) Benign breast disease and cancer. *Br. J. Surg., 67,* 789–790.

Dupont, W.D. & Page, D.L. (1985) Risk factors for breast cancer in women with proliferative breast disease. *N. Engl. J. Med., 312,* 146–151.

Foote, F.W. & Stewart, F.W. (1941) Lobular carcinoma in situ: a rare form of mammary cancer. *Am. J. Path., 17,* 491–495.

Haagensen, C.D., Lane, N., Lattes, R. & Bodian, C. (1978) Lobular neoplasia (so called lobular carcinoma in situ) of the breast. *Cancer, 42,* 737–769.

Harris, J.R., Connolly, J., Schnitt, S.J., Cohen, R.B. & Hellman, S. (1983) Clinical-pathological study of early breast cancer treated by primary radiation therapy. *J. Clin. Oncol., 1,* 184–189.

McDivitt, R.W., Stewart, F.W. & Berg, J.W. (1968) Tumours of the breast. *Armed Forces Institute of Pathology Atlas of Tumour Pathology,* Second Series, Part 2. Washington D.C.

Page, D.L., Vander, Swaag R., Rogers, L.W. et al (1978) Relation between component parts of fibrocystic disease complex and breast cancer. *J. Nat. Cancer Inst., 62,* 641–709.

Page, D.L., Dupont, W.E., Rogers, L.W. & Rados, M.S. (1985) Atypical hyperlastic lesions of the female breast: a long term follow-up study. *Cancer* (in press).

Warren, S. (1940) The relationship of 'chronic mastitis' to carcinoma of the breast. *Surg. Gynecol. Obstet., 71,* 257–273.

Wellings, S.R. (1976) Persistent and atypical lobules in the human breast may be precancerous. *Experientia, 32,* 1463–1465.

3 Lesions which May be Mistaken for Breast Carcinoma

Christopher Elston and Roger Blamey

In the last chapter we discussed the difficult area in the borderline between benign and malignant disease. This chapter is concerned with lesions which, although inherently benign, have features which may lead to an incorrect diagnosis of carcinoma. We have divided them into two groups: a group where the main diagnostic difficulty is encountered histopathologically and where mammographic features also cause problems (indeed, the increase in the use of mammography, especially in screening programmes, leads to an increased number of such lesions), and a group where the difficulties are essentially clinical.

Histological and mammographic difficulties

Radial scar A number of different terms have been applied to the distinctive sclerosing epithelial lesion in the breast that is now called a radial scar. These include 'sclerosing papillary proliferation', 'Strahlige Narben', 'benign sclerosing ductal proliferation' and 'infiltrating epitheliosis' (Azzopardi, 1979).

Morphologically, radial scars, as the name implies, consist of radiating stellate tissue with a dense central fibroelastolic core (Fig. 3.1). They range in size between 5 and 10 mm. Within the arms of the stellate configuration, ducts and lobules appear to be drawn into the centre of the lesion by the contraction of the elastolic tissue. Some of the epithelial structures are cystically dilated (Fig. 3.2) and epithelial proliferation (epitheliosis) is frequently present, with or without atypia.

At one time radial scars were thought to be rare, but extensive studies have now shown that they are relatively common and often multiple (Linell et al, 1980). They appear to be part of the spectrum of changes seen in benign mammary dysplasia, but the reason for the sclerosing nature of the lesion must remain a matter for speculation.

Radial scar may cause diagnostic difficulty in two respects. The radiating stellate configuration may closely mimic the appearances of a carcinoma on mammography (Chapter 8) although now that the lesion is becoming better recognized experienced radiologists can usually distinguish the two processes. Of greater importance is the fact that radial scar may be mistaken for a

Figure 3.1
Radial scar. Dilated
ducts are drawn into
a central elastolic core
in a stellate
fashion. H&E ×8.

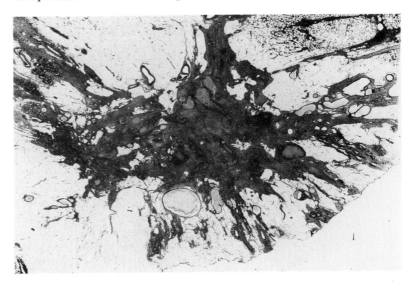

tubular carcinoma histologically. In most cases the distinction
should be relatively simple. In a radial scar the epithelium is
regular and both epithelial and myoepithelial cells are apparent.
There is no nuclear atypia and mitoses are extremely rare.
Occasionally more florid epithelial proliferation is seen and the
appearances may approach those of in-situ carcinoma. The
presence of other manifestations of mammary dysplasia such as
duct dilatation, pink cell change, and sclerosing adenosis,
further help to distinguish radial scar from tubular carcinoma.

Figure 3.2
Higher power view of
Figure 3.1 showing
dilated ducts and
solid tubules.
H&E ×120.

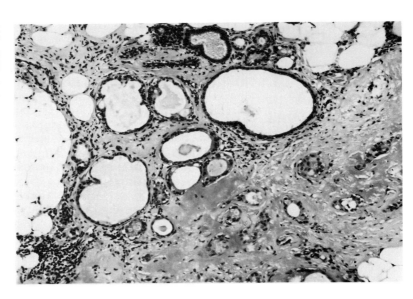

Figure 3.3
Sclerosing adenosis.
There is a disorderly
proliferation of epi-
thelial, myoepithelial
and stromal cells,
with some open
tubules. Note the
microcalcification
(arrowed).
H&E ×290.

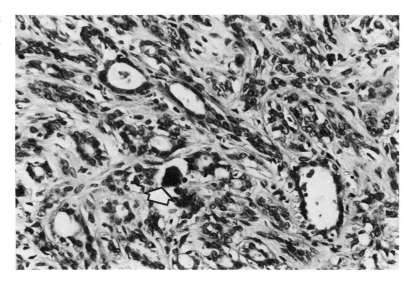

The status of radial scar as a premalignant lesion is disputed. Linell et al (1980) have argued strongly in favour of a progression from radial scar to tubular carcinoma, and that the latter are the source for many infiltrating ductal carcinomas. Their evidence is at best circumstantial and cannot be regarded as conclusive, while other workers believe that radial scars are entirely benign (Azzopardi, 1979). On balance, the current evidence suggests that radial scars are benign, with a very low risk of subsequent carcinoma. If they are treated by local excision because their mammographic appearance mimics cancer, then long-term follow-up is unnecessary.

Sclerosing adenosis

While the term 'adenosis' is grossly overused in breast pathology 'sclerosing adenosis' describes a specific proliferative lesion of the terminal duct–lobular unit. It may occur as part of the spectrum of mammary dysplasia, or as a nodular tumour-like mass in an otherwise normal breast, especially in younger women. Macroscopically, the lesion tends to have an ill-defined multinodular appearance. The tissue is firm but rarely as hard as a carcinoma. Microscopically, there is a disorderly epithelial and myoepithelial proliferation in which the regular outline of the lobules is lost (Fig. 3.3). A whorled configuration of tubules is often seen, but luminal structures may be indistinct. The tubules are lined by both epithelial and myoepithelial cells of regular appearance without nuclear atypia. Mitoses are infrequent. At the periphery of nodules an increased amount of stromal prolifer-ation is seen, with varying degrees of sclerosis. Foci of microcal-cification are frequently seen within tubular structures.

As with radial scar, sclerosing adenosis may be confused with carcinoma in two respects. The microcalcification when seen on

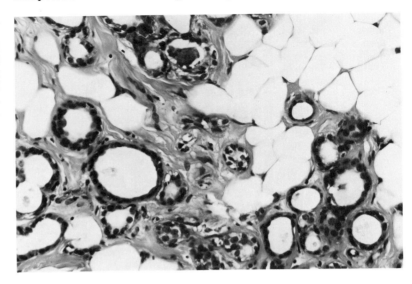

Figure 3.4
Microglandular ade-
nosis. Small open and
solid tubules extend
in an irregular fashion
into connective and
adipose tissue.
H&E ×290.

a mammogram (Chapter 8) is virtually indistinguishable from an intraduct carcinoma, except by the most experienced radiologist. It follows that when a mammographic diagnosis of malignancy is based on the finding of microcalcification, excision biopsy is often performed to confirm the diagnosis. The second, and more important area of diagnostic difficulty, is histological. The poorly circumscribed disorderly epithelial proliferation may be mistaken for invasive carcinoma, especially by inexperienced pathologists. The most useful distinguishing feature is the fact that the tubules of sclerosing adenosis are lined by two layers of cells, epithelial and myoepithelial, while carcinomatous tubules are made up of a single cell layer. In well fixed and processed material, diagnostic difficulty should occur only rarely, but genuine problems may be encountered with frozen section or Trucut biopsy. If the pathologist has any doubt in such circumstances, a benign report should be issued and definitive paraffin blocks examined.

The management of patients in whom a diagnosis of sclerosing adenosis is made is straightforward. The lesion does not carry an increased risk of subsequent carcinoma (Dupont and Page, 1985) and local excision without further follow-up is sufficient treatment.

*Microglandular
adenosis*

This is the term which has been applied to an uncommon lesion in which there is an ill-defined proliferation of small glandular structures into connective and adipose tissue (Clement and Azzopardi, 1983). It tends to occur in the perimenopausal age group and while it may be seen as part of benign mammary dysplasia, it can form palpable masses clinically similar to a carcinoma. The lesion may be unifocal or multifocal. Histologically, it consists of poorly circumscribed proliferations of small glands which appear to infiltrate the stroma and adipose tissue in unstructured formation (Fig. 3.4). At the margins of the lesion an association with adjacent normal lobules is sometimes apparent. The glandular tubules mostly have clear rounded laminae although solid epithelial structures do occur. They are usually lined by a single layer of epithelial cells, and myoepithelial cells are not seen. Nuclei are small and regular without atypia or mitoses.

Microglandular adenosis does not cause diagnostic difficulty clinically, and there are no mammographic features which mimic a malignant process. Histologically, however, it may be mistaken for a tubular carcinoma, especially because the tubules are lined only by a single layer of cells. Clement and Azzopardi (1983) have discussed the distinguishing features fully and only the more important points will be mentioned here. The glands in microglandular adenosis are more regular in outline than a tubular carcinoma and appear to infiltrate more diffusely, epithelial apical 'snouts' typical of tubular carcinoma are not seen, and the nuclei have no features to suggest malignancy. In tubular carcinoma the stroma is desmoplastic and elastotic, often with central scarring, while the stroma in microglandular adenosis is inconspicuous and often composed of adipose tissue alone. Management of microglandular adenosis is straightforward. The lesion is entirely benign, and in our view has some similarities with sclerosing adenosis. Although the number of cases reported is small there is no evidence to suggest that the lesion conveys an increased risk of subsequent carcinoma. Follow-up is therefore not required.

Adenoma of the nipple This uncommon lesion of the nipple ducts has been given a number of synonyms, including 'subareolar duct papillomatosis' (McDivitt et al, 1968), but adenoma of the nipple is now the preferred term (Azzopardi, 1979).

The lesion may occur at any age, but is most common in the fourth and fifth decades. It normally presents as nipple discharge which may be bloodstained, and on examination the nipple is indurated, reddened and often crusted. The duration of symptoms varies from a few weeks to several years. Clinically, adenoma of the nipple is indistinguishable from Paget's disease of the nipple, which is naturally the commonest preoperative diagnosis.

Macroscopically, the lesion forms a relatively well circumscribed nodule in the nipple and areolar area which may appear to ulcerate the overlying epidermis. Microscopically (Fig. 3.5), the edges of the nodule are not sharply defined and tend to merge with adjacent normal ducts. There is a florid proliferation of tubules in which both epithelial and myoepithelial cells can be identified. The cells are uniform in size and shape without nuclear atypia and although mitoses may be found they are not abnormal. In some cases epithelial proliferation may be pro-

Figure 3.5
Adenoma of nipple.
The nipple epithelium
is ulcerated at the top
right by an underlying
glandular prolifera-
tion. H&E ×120.

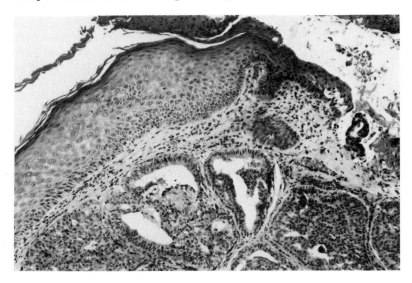

nounced and resemble epitheliosis with solid tubular structures. There is a variable amount of stroma and a papillary pattern may be discerned, especially close to the epidermis. There is no doubt that before adenoma of the nipple was formally described (Jones, 1955) cases were mistaken for well differentiated ductal or tubular carcinoma. The great majority of these tumours are now known to be benign (Azzopardi, 1979) and the histopathologist must assess each case with care. The presence of two-layered epithelium, and the lack of nuclear atypia are clear points in favour of a benign lesion. Very rare cases of carcinomatous change in nipple adenoma have been recorded, but the microscopical features of malignancy were present in the lesions (Azzopardi, 1979).

Adenoma of the nipple should be managed by complete local excision. While this may appear drastic for a benign condition, attempts to preserve the nipple may lead to unsightly deformity, with the risk of incomplete excision.

Clinical difficulties

Phyllodes tumour   This tumour usually presents after the age of 50. It often gives rise to a large, smooth, bosselated lump in the breast, sometimes seeming to occupy the whole breast. The obvious diagnosis of a large mass in the breast is carcinoma; this tumour is, however, mobile, attaching neither to skin nor to deep tissues and rarely ulcerating through the skin (which it achieves by necrosis and not by invasion).

Macroscopically, the cut surface has a characteristic whorled and nodular pattern reminiscent of a leaf bud (*phylos*, Gk = leaf). Microscopically (Fig. 3.6), the tumour is composed of irregular clefts lined by epithelial cells set in a cellular fibroblastic stroma.

Figure 3.6
Phyllodes tumour.
Note the epithelium-
lined cleft and the
cellular stoma.
H&E ×78.

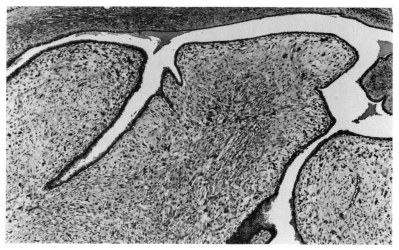

Since the tumour is usually benign, complete local excision is carried out. If the patient is elderly and the tumour is very large they may prefer to undergo mastectomy.

In a minority of cases, histological examination shows that the stroma has undergone sarcomatous change. In such cases, rapid local recurrence may occur and repeat operation, with wide local excision including underlying muscle, is required to prevent this. In cases where the tumour proves sarcomatous, rapid recurrence may occur and wide excision is then mandatory.

Fat necrosis

Fat necrosis, too, is a disease of the fifth and sixth decades. It may present as a lump with skin tether or as a lump with surrounding bruising. There is often no history of trauma. The lesion presumably reflects greater blood vessel fragility at this age. In younger women the lesion may present with a clear history of trauma, for instance a blow from the steering wheel in a motor accident.

The diagnosis is made by Trucut needle biopsy. This is one of the exceptions to the rule that a solid lump must always be removed for full histological examination if the Trucut does not show carcinoma (Chapter 1). A good history of the physical signs of bruising, accompanied by the histological confirmation of haematoma or fat necrosis, can be accepted. If there is no such history but these features are present on Trucut biopsy, then we prefer to follow the lump until it has resolved clinically and then ensure that there is no mammographic abnormality.

Breast abscess

Breast abscess is not infrequent outside the puerperium but is almost always restricted to premenopausal women. The clinical features, as might be expected, are those of redness, heat, and the extreme tenderness of the lump.

Figure 3.7
Adenosis of pregnancy. The lobules are hyperplastic with dilated acini containing secretion.
H&E ×126.

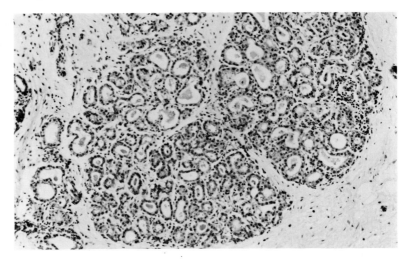

As with fat necrosis, Trucut biopsy is used to confirm the clinical diagnosis (after the extreme tenderness has gone out of the lump) and resolution is awaited. Again, resolution should be complete clinically and mammographically or excision biopsy must be carried out. Carcinoma presenting as an acute abscess has in fact been rare in our series.

Not infrequently, a breast abscess will be seen as a non-tender lump in the referral clinic. History then reveals that the features were as above but antibiotics given by the patient's general practitioner, had removed the inflammation. If the history is very clear, then management is as above, but if there is any doubt and the Trucut biopsy shows no carcinoma, then the lump must be removed for full histological examination.

Adenosis of pregnancy

Adenosis of pregnancy is the usual name given to a palpable lump occurring in pregnancy. The clinical presentation is of a lump— usually large, 5–6 cm in diameter—presenting at any stage of the pregnancy from three months on, or even in early lactation. The lump is clearly defined from the surrounding breast tissue even though there is general engorgement. Histologically (Fig. 3.7), the appearances are those of entirely normal, hyperplastic breast tissue, indistinguishable from the remainder of the breast. The lesion is probably no more than an exaggeration of the physiological hyperplasia of normal pregnancy. The term 'adenoma' of pregnancy has been applied to this condition and is a misnomer.

Our management is to take Trucut biopsies from both ends of the lump and repeat these after two weeks. If these biopsies show only the appearances described above, then the patient remains under observation at six weekly intervals, until the lump settles after parturition and lactation.

Controversies
and Future
Developments

• Greater mammographic expertise to avoid unnecessary biopsies. Again, specialist breast clinics are a prerequisite.

References

Azzopardi, J.G. (1979) *Problems in Breast Pathology* [For radial scar, pp. 174–187; For adenosis of nipple, pp. 260–266]. London: W.B. Saunders.

Clement, P.B. & Azzopardi, J.G. (1983) Microglandular adenosis of the breast—a lesion simulating tubular carcinoma. *Histopathology, 7,* 169–180.

Dupont, W.D. & Page, D.L. (1985) Risk factors for breast cancer in women with proliferative breast disease. *New Engl. J. Med., 312,* 146–151.

Jones, D.B. (1955) Florid papillomatosis of the nipple ducts. *Cancer, 8,* 315–319.

Linell, F., Ljungberg, O. & Andersson, I. (1980) Breast carcinoma—aspects of early stages, progression and related problems. *Acta Pathol. Microbiol. Scand. [A] [Suppl. 272].*

McDivitt, R.W., Stewart, F.W. & Berg, J.W. (1968) Tumours of the breast. *Armed Forces Institute of Pathology Atlas of Tumour Pathology,* Second Series, Part 2, pp. 138–143. Washington D.C.

4 Nipple Discharge and Duct Ectasia

Howard Holliday and Christopher Hinton

Nipple Discharge

Between 5 and 10% of referrals to breast clinics and well-women units are for nipple discharge, the majority being young premenopausal women. This chapter will concentrate on the management of women who have a nipple discharge in the absence of a lump. Our figures show that only about 4% of women with a nipple discharge have breast cancer.

A significant nipple discharge is a spontaneous discharge; discharge as a result of manual expresson is unimportant and can be elicited in up to 50% of premenopausal women. Spontaneous discharge may occur in certain physiological or endocrine situations such as menstruation, pregnancy, in association with drug intake (psychotropics, antihypertensives, oral contraceptives) and in hyperprolactinaemic states. Persistent lactation and galactorrhoea may be effectively due to hyperprolactinaemia but in practice it is rare to find prolactin-secreting microadenomas of the pituitary. If not due to an endocrine disorder, nipple discharge indicates a pathological change within the breast. Pathological discharges tend to be intermittent and commonly from a single duct, whilst physiological discharges are bilateral and multiduct in origin. The main causes of a single duct nipple discharge are duct ectasia, mammary dysplasia, intraduct papilloma, intraduct carcinoma and invasive carcinoma.

Management

A relevant history is taken to indicate possible drug usage and endocrine disorders. It is interesting to record the nature of the discharge but this is in no way diagnostic. Bloody and serous discharge can occur in both cancer and dysplasia (Funderburk and Syphax, 1969) and most patients with a blood-stained nipple discharge do not have cancer.

The two prime objectives of examination are to detect any lumps in the breast and to identify the duct or ducts from which the discharge issues. If a lump is detected then the management of the patient becomes the management of that breast lump. The remainder of this chapter assumes that the problem is of discharge in the absence of lump. In the absence of a lump the nipple is carefully inspected as pressure is applied around the areola. Usually pressure close to the areola will elicit a discharge and the site and number of discharging ducts should be accurately recorded in the notes.

Cytological examination of the discharge cannot be completely relied upon for a diagnosis but is an aid to diagnosis (with the same reservations as discussed in Chapter 1). Normal cytology cannot be taken as indicating an absence of malignancy.

Further assessment of the breast is made by mammography. Plain mammography is considered totally unhelpful by some. In Nottingham we have found mammography accurate in the detection of the two cancers among the 52 women who had mammography for nipple discharge in the absence of a palpable lump. Tabar et al (1983) had a 100% success rate demonstrating cancers by ductography, but all these patients had single duct discharge only and they did not claim that normal ductography would erradicate the need for biopsy. Ductography is a fairly simple technique whereby a small amount of contrast medium is injected into the discharging duct and displayed by mammography (Chapter 8, Fig. 8.3).

Multiduct discharge

In the absence of a lump or mammographic abnormality, the number of discharging ducts is noted. A multiduct discharge indicates diffuse breast disease, is often bilateral and is therefore extremely unlikely to be caused by cancer—it would be unusual for a tumour to involve more than one duct system and not demonstrate any clinical signs. Multiduct discharge in the absence of a lump immediately precludes cancer; mammography makes this decision even easier.

A patient with troublesome multiduct discharge causing social embarrassment should have a prolactin estimation. Prolactin-secreting pituitary adenomas are rare, but if found the nipple discharge may be treated using bromocriptine. Otherwise, the patient can be cured of discharge if symptoms warrant, by complete duct disconnection through a circumareolar incision.

Single duct discharge

Single duct discharge, in the absence of lump or mammographic abnormality, is investigated by the operation of microdochectomy (Atkins and Wolff, 1964). This operation may be carried out under local or general anaesthetic. A fine ophthalmic probe is introduced into the duct in question, the duct is isolated, and is then completely excised.

We detected 4 cancers in 73 women with single duct discharge (Table 4.1). Thirty-one other women had a distinct pathological entity, intraduct papilloma (Fig. 4.1), to account for their discharge. Haagensen (1971) does not consider intraduct papilloma to be premalignant and we agree. There is now no need for speculative blind mastectomy to be performed for every case of nipple discharge. This was previously advocated by Atkins for women over 45 years with haemoccult-positive discharge, and

	Single duct discharge	*Multiduct discharge*
Duct ectasia	26	3
Intraduct papilloma	31	23
Mammary dysplasia	12	1
Intraduct carcinoma	4	

Seltzer et al (1970) recommended mastectomy for any woman over 60 years with a discharge. Older women are certainly more at risk, but there is no need to stray from the policy defined above.

The intermittent nature of nipple discharge frequently results in no abnormality being detected in the out-patient clinic and a repeat examination is therefore recommended. Failure to elicit a discharge is not significant and those who cease to discharge do so without ill effect. This is a common occurrence in premenopausal women.

A patient may complain of nipple discharge where, in fact, inversion has resulted in superficial accumulation of fluid. A careful history will resolve this situation. Crusting on the nipple surface due to a discharge is usually easily removed and so distinguished from Paget's disease.

Where there is discharge after previous microdochectomy, review of the initial pathology may indicate that further discharge is not sinister and could be anticipated, e.g. in the presence of duct ectasia. However, if the previous diagnosis showed intraduct papilloma, these may be multiple. This should result in careful follow-up of the patient and further biopsy,

Figure 4.1
Duct papilloma. The ductal lumen contains an intraduct papilloma lined by benign epithelial cells. H&E ×315.

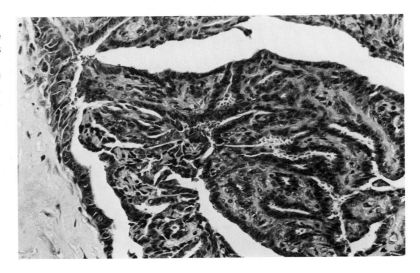

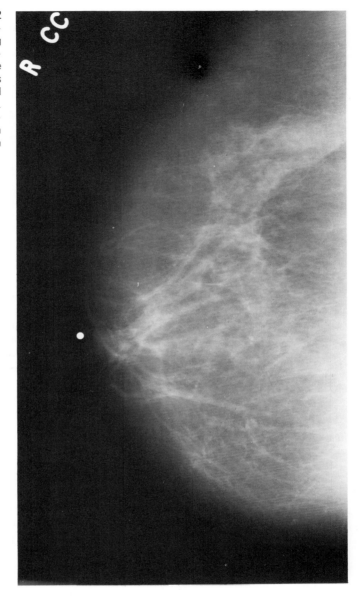

probably excision of the central ducts by removal of the subareolar part of the breast.

Conclusion
Nipple discharge is a worrisome condition for patient and
clinician. However, it can be managed by a simple protocol.
Biopsy is indicated for an associated mass or mammographic

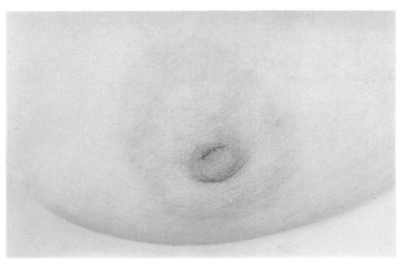

abnormality. Microdochectomy is carried out for single duct discharge. Bloody discharge is not synonymous with cancer, and a clear discharge does not indicate benignity. For persistent bilateral discharge, prolactin levels are taken, and the pituitary fossa imaged; treatment for this condition with bromocriptine may be helpful. Symptomatic multiduct discharge can be relieved by duct excision.

Duct ectasia

Duct ectasia is a condition in which the ducts immediately under the nipple are dilated. It is a frequent cause of nipple discharge (Table 4.1) and may be seen mammographically (Fig. 4.2). In addition, the duct may harbour infection and give rise to recurrent, rather indolent, painful abscesses, lying within or close to the areola. In the face of recurrent abscesses, an operation removing the central breast tissue under the areola is carried out by means of an incision running around the lower edge of the areola, disconnecting the nipple. The incision into the breast tissue is cut to a depth of around 2–3 cm so that all the central duct system is removed from below the areola.

The Indrawn Nipple

It is well recognized and widely stressed in student teaching that nipple retraction can be one of the first signs of breast cancer. What is less well recognized is the fact that in the majority of cases nipple retraction is benign.

Longstanding nipple inversion arising at puberty or during pregnancy and lactation is always benign and is easily recog-

Figure 4.4
Nipple indrawn by
underlying carcinoma.

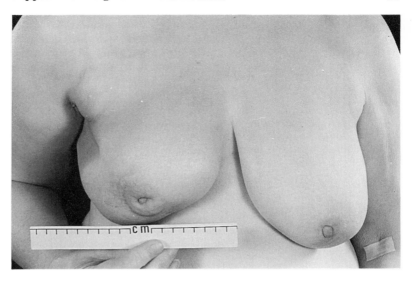

nized (Fig. 4.3). Characteristically it is bilateral (though not invariably) with a significant slit-like appearance and with no deformity of the areola or surrounding skin. It is not associated with any specific disease process in the breast. Diagnostic difficulty arises in women who present, usually in their fifties to seventies, with recent indrawing of the nipple. Although most cases are benign it is in this group that carcinoma must be sought. Mammary duct ectasia is the most common pathological cause of indrawing of the nipple presenting to a breast clinic. The appearances of the nipple in this condition are commonly like those of the longstanding inversion described above but may progress to a picture of retraction of the whole nipple with accompanying dilation of the areola and surrounding skin. The process is caused by fibrosis around the ectatic ducts which contract and shorten leading to a gradual indrawing of the nipple, usually from the centre.

By contrast, the nipple retraction due to carcinoma is a result of involvement of the breast ducts by the tumour resulting in their distortion. The tumour is commonly to one side producing tilting and distortion of the nipple towards the tumour as a result of the pulling of the ducts in that direction (Fig. 4.4).

The management of patients presenting with an indrawn nipple

When a patient presents to a breast clinic with an indrawn nipple the correct diagnosis can in almost all cases be made by careful history-taking and examination. The length of history and circumstances of onset are of great importance. Points of importance in the examination helping to exclude a diagnosis of cancer are the appearance of the nipple, the ability to evert the nipple, the presence of palpable ectatic ducts felt as cord beneath the nipple when rolled between the examiner's fingers, and, of course, the absence of a lump. Mammography is carried out as the final investigation to exclude a carcinoma in the retroareolar region.

Treatment is in most cases unnecessary.

Controversies and Future Developments

• With carcinoma-in-situ the underlying cause of single duct discharge in 5% of cases and the majority of these visible mammographically, is microdochectomy now outdated?

References

Atkins, H. & Wolff, B. (1964) Discharge from the nipple. *Br. J. Surg.*, *51*, 602–606.

Funderburk, W.W. & Syphax, B. (1969) Evaluation of nipple discharge in benign and malignant diseases. *Cancer*, *24*, 1290–1296.

Haagensen, C.D. (1971) *Diseases of the Breast*. London: W.B. Saunders.

Seltzer, M.H., Perloff, L.J., Kelley, R.I. & Fitts, L.T. (1970) The significance of age in patients with nipple discharge. *Surg. Gynecol. Obstet.*, *131*, 519–522.

Tabar, L., Dean, P.B. & Pentek, Z. (1983) Galactography: the diagnostic procedure of choice for nipple discharge. *Radiology*, *149*, 31–38.

Urban, J. (1978) Non lactatical nipple discharge. *Cancer*, *28(3)*, 130–140.

5 The Early Detection of Breast Cancer

Roger Blamey

Screening for breast cancer relies on the argument that prognosis correlates with size of the tumour and lymph node involvement. These observations do not prove the case; for example the relationship might come about because slow-growing tumours remain small for some time. Possibly all breast cancers have metastasized before reaching the size at which screening programmes can detect them.

The New York Health Insurance Plan (HIP) trial (Shapiro et al, 1981) involved screening 31 000 women and at the same time 31 000 women were identified but were not offered screening. Allocation was random, the age span 40–64 years, and the method of screening was invitation to four annual clinical and mammographic examinations.

Five years from the time of entry of all woman to the study, there was a one-third reduction in mortality from breast cancer in the study group as against the controls (Table 5.1). A reduction in mortality is maintained to the present time, 13 years from the start of the trial.

This reduction in mortality was achieved in the total study group, which includes women invited for screening but who did not attend (only 65% came for the first screening, and only 50% attended all four). The figures at 13 years include cases diagnosed well after the period of study.

Recently a multicentre controlled trial in Sweden (Tabar et al, 1985), published seven years after commencement, has given a similar result. The similarity extends to the fact that the proven benefit in both trials is restricted to women over the age of 50. This result in the HIP study was thought to reflect the denseness of the premenopausal breast and the relatively lower resolution of the mammograms some years ago during the HIP study. The overall result of these trials, showing a lowering in mortality from breast cancer in the group invited for screening, is of great importance and powerful evidence for the beneficial effect of screening.

Further examination of the effect is made by consideration of case fatality rate (CFR). Before examining CFR, it is important to ensure that there is no diagnosis of spurious cancer in the study group. The number of cancers diagnosed in the HIP study by the end of the initial five year period (up to an average of 18 months

Table 5.1
Deaths from breast
cancer in the
controlled trials.

		5 years	9 years	13 years
HIP	Study group	39	70	116
	Control group	63	108	148
Sweden	Study group	87	(population at risk = 78 085)	
	Control group	86	(population at risk = 56 782)	

after screening ended) was 303 in the Study Group (2 per 1000 patient years) and 293 in the Control (1.9 per 1000 patient years). These are sufficiently close for us to conclude that all cases diagnosed as cancer in the study group would have progressed to clinical cancer.

Study of the cumulative CFR in the HIP study show, as might be expected, that the cancers diagnosed through screening (132 of the 303 study group cancers) had the best prognosis with a five year survival of 87% (compare with Chapter 7) and an 11 year survival of 72%. The cancers presenting between screenings in those women who had attended screening (interval cancers), and the cancers presenting in women invited for screening but not attending, had the same prognosis as the control group: these three groups had five year survival between 60 and 65% and 11 year survivals between 44 and 46%. The similarity of outcome of these latter three groups, and the comparison with the group of cancers detected at screening, is strong argument that the reduction in mortality of the study group was achieved by early detection at the screening examinations.

These trials are the firmest evidence that screening can reduce mortality from breast cancer. Two case control studies from Holland suggest that screening can half the risk of dying from breast cancer over a six year period.

The search for cost-effectiveness

Annual mammographic screening is extremely expensive. Since it appears that only 1 woman in 4 has a cancer which is altered by screening, it would cost around £50 000 per annum to ameliorate the course of one cancer.

An obvious approach is the use of predictive factors to identify a small group of women who will produce the majority of breast cancers and who alone would then be screened. Unfortunately neither epidemiological nor hormonal factors (Vessey, 1981), alone or in combination, are powerful enough to produce a reasonable equation (this would have to be in the region of 80% of all breast cancers occurring in an identifiable 25% of all women aged 40 years or over).

Mammography is a technically efficient method of detecting breast abnormalities. Other physical methods, such as ultrasound, may ultimately prove to be as effective, but since all necessitate operator salaries the cost of any physical method is likely to be similar to the cost of mammography.

The Swedish study used only single oblique views for their mammograms and carried these out only every 2–3 years. Clinical examinations carried out by nurse or doctor can be omitted since I believe that they are totally ineffective. From personal experience I know that I could not find the one necessary 1 cm lump in 2000 breasts consecutively palpated.

Breast self-examination

For ultimate cheapness in Nottingham we are evaluating Education on Breast Self-Examination (B.S.E.) and Self-Referral as part of the D.H.S.S. study of early detection.

The theory behind this is more encouraging than an initial statement of the project might suggest. From clinical experience, women examining themselves certainly can detect breast lumps at a small size (around 1 cm). The typical case of this, which all surgeons will recognize, is the young woman with a small fibroadenoma: it is not easy for the surgeon to locate this until the woman herself puts her finger on it and then it is easily felt. In comparison, the majority of cases detected in mammographic programmes are at the 0.5 to 1 cm size. The size of a tumour is closely related to node involvement, thus a diminution of size at detection will result in more tumours without node involvement.

Present recommendations regarding early detection of breast cancer

The evidence, stated above, is that mammographic screening is beneficial. Anyone seeking advice regardless of personal cost should be recommended annual mammography from the age of 40.

A woman with a mother, grandmother or sister who has breast cancer, has a substantially increased chance of herself contracting breast cancer; around 10% of breast cancer patients will have such a history. A woman who has had a breast biopsy showing cellular atypia may similarly have an increased chance of breast cancer (Chapter 2). The combination of atypia and family history is particularly important. A woman who has had primary breast cancer treated and appears to have a good prognosis, has a greatly increased chance of breast cancer arising in the opposite breast in subsequent years—around 1% per annum. All these three groups should receive annual mammography.

For the majority of women at the present time screening is a promising method of detection but not fully proven and not freely available. For these women a recommendation to examine themselves would appear to do little harm. The establishment of an education programme in this direction and of self-referral clinics for women to attend if they discover an apparent abnormality, would be an encouragement.

The future of screening for breast cancer

The benefit of screening is becoming accepted. A cost-effective method of screening will have to be found. This may prove to be a combination of using mammography triennially, by a single oblique view method without clinical examination, to pick up those cancers (perhaps 20%) which have a long in-situ phase before invasion, backed up by education in self-palpation and self-referral, aimed at the initially invasive and more rapidly growing tumours.

Use of the present screening methods may be temporary and may be replaced by scientific research aimed at detection of either the presence of breast cancer, by examination of serum antigen levels, or detection of the predisposition to breast cancer by DNA analysis, once the genes coding for breast cancer has been identified and analysed.

Further reading

Shapiro, S., Venet, W., Strax, P., Venet, L. & Roeser, R. (1982) Ten to fourteen year effects of breast cancer screening on mortality. *J.N.C.I.,* *69,* 349–355.

Tabar, L., Fagerberg, C.J.G., Gad, A. et al (1985) Reduction in mortality from breast cancer after mass screening with mammography *Lancet, i,* 829–832.

Vessey, M. (1981) A review of the risk factors. *Reviews on Endocrine-related Cancer, Suppl. 10,* 41.

6 Early Detection of Breast Cancer by Breast Self-Examination

Christopher Hinton

In 1979 the Department of Health and Social Security set up in the United Kingdom a trial of Early Detection of Breast Cancer to look at the efficacy and cost of different methods of early breast cancer detection. They chose to evaluate two methods of early detection: (1) annual clinical examination with mammography in alternate years, and (2) an intensive programme of education in breast self-examination. Each of these means of early detection are being tested in two health districts and four further health districts have been selected as control areas, so that these early detection methods can be compared with conventional diagnostic services in the National Health Service. Nottingham is involved in a programme of education in breast self-examination.

The Nottingham programme has involved the invitation of every woman between the ages of 45 and 65 living in the South Nottingham Health District to a talk and film on breast self-examination and the provision of a self-referral unit where women may subsequently come if they think they have found an abnormality in the breast.

It is far too early to draw any conclusions on the influence of the self-examination programme on mortality from breast cancer but encouraging changes have been seen in the characteristics of the tumours presenting in Nottingham over the period of the study. The proportion of tumours presenting in an advanced, inoperable state, has been halved—from 27%, prior to the introducton of the education programme, to 13% afterwards. Among operable tumours there has been a marked trend towards patients presenting with smaller tumours such that now almost 60% of patients present with tumours of 2 cm or less (Fig. 6.1) and the proportion of patients found to have axillary nodal involvement at mastectomy has been reduced from 52% to 35%. These findings give hope that a reduction in mortality from the disease will follow but it will be many years before this is known.

Problems
Any programme of intervention aimed at early detection of disease has some problems associated with it and a programme of breast self-examination is no exception. These problems can

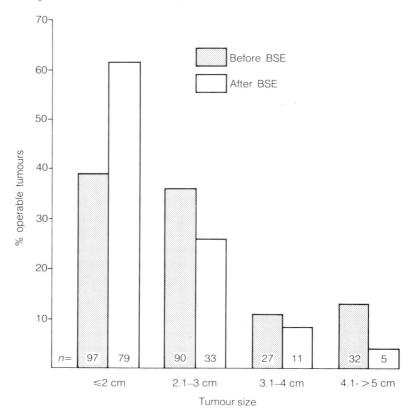

Figure 6.1
Distribution of
tumour size (operable
cancers) (a) before
BSE: women between
45 and 64 presenting
1974–79; (b) after
BSE: women in the
study group
(attenders and non-
attenders). (Figure
reproduced from
Blamey, R.W., 1984.
Breast Cancer,
London. Update
Publications.)

broadly be divided into two categories: (1) those associated with any programme of early detection of breast cancer, and (2) those complications relating specifically to a programme of breast self-examination.

General complications of early detection schemes in breast cancer as applied to a programme of breast self-examination

Attendance

For a programme of early detection of breast cancer to have any chance of success it is first necessary for women to attend the sessions—in this case for education in breast self-examination.

Experience in the Nottingham scheme suggests that the method by which the invitation is issued is of considerable importance to the rate of acceptance of the invitation.

In the early days of the scheme women were not approached directly, but rather by means of advertising both in the local press and by leaflet distribution. These attempts failed almost totally. Subsequently, women were sent personal invitations by letter. In some areas these letters were sent direct from the breast-screening unit. This form of invitation has resulted in attendance rates of approximately 35%. In other areas, the invitation to the talk and film took the form of a personal letter to each woman from her General Practitioner. In response to this form of invitation, over 50% of those women invited attended the classes. It seems, therefore, that women are more likely to attend if the invitation comes from someone that she knows and to whom she can personally relate.

If this form of invitation is to be used, it is essential to recruit the cooperation of the local general practitioners from the outset. If women are being approached on an individual basis it is important to avoid where possible the distress which may be caused by issuing such an invitation to a woman who has already been treated for breast cancer, or worse, to someone who has recently died of the disease. To minimize the possibility of this, lists have been sent to general practitioners of women in their practice who are to be invited to be checked against their records.

An attendance rate of 50% may seem disappointing, but attempts to increase this by subsequent reinvitation have not proved rewarding. Issuing second invitations to women who have failed to attend in response to their first invitation has resulted in attendance rates of less than 10%.

There are a number of reasons for the apparently disappointing rate of attendance. The accuracy of the initial list is important as is the accuracy of the information it provides. Regular updating of the information is vital, particularly with regard to address changes. Estimates of the accuracy of the list as supplied by us by comparison with other records such as the electoral register and census surveys, have suggested an error rate of at least 18% and possibly more. It should also not be forgotten that information for breast self-examination is available through other sources, particularly the press, and that women who already examine their breasts are unlikely to come to be taught again.

For these reasons it seems that attendance rates in the order of 50% are likely to be the best that can reasonably be expected for this type of scheme.

The management of abnormalities

If a programme of breast self-examination is to work, then women who attend a lecture and talk on breast self-examination must be able to detect abnormalities in their breasts which they would otherwise not have detected at that time. In the initial period, therefore, there is inevitably an increase in the number of women seeking advice about abnormalities, which may or may not be significant, in their breasts. In addition, it is to be hoped that they will become experts at examining their own breasts and will be able to detect changes which might not, even to a trained examiner, be readily apparent. In the absence of special provisions, the burden of determining abnormality falls on the shoulders of the G.P. who may have no special interest or training in breast disease.

To try to overcome these difficulties a self-referral unit has been provided for women in the South Nottingham scheme. In order to keep costs to a minimum, this unit is staffed by specially trained nurses who have been able to develop some expertise in breast palpation over a prolonged period of training in the hospital breast clinics. The procedure allows a woman attending the self-referral clinic to be seen and examined by one of these nurses and mammography is performed as an additional check. The mammogram is, in the first instance, read by a radiographer who has been specially trained in the interpretation of mammography. If both the nurse and the radiographer agree that there is no detectable abnormality, the patient is discharged without consultation with medical staff. If there appears to be any abnormality or there is doubt regarding either examination, then a consultation with the clinic doctor (a surgeon with a special interest in breast disease) is arranged. In this way the number of secondary consultations presenting to local general practitioners or to hospital breast clinics are kept to a minimum.

An important question which must be answered is: is this policy of women being examined by nursing staff and mammography interpreted by radiographers safe? In the first three years of the Nottingham self-examination programme, 1295 patients were seen on the self-referral unit. Six hundred and ninety-six patients were discharged at the time of the first examination without consultation with medical staff. In none of these patients, with a minium follow-up of one year, has cancer been detected. This confirms the ability of nursing staff to differentiate accurately normal from abnormal, which, in practice, is all that they are asked to do.

Benign breast disease
There are two aspects of benign breast disease which are important to programmes of early detection in breast cancer. Firstly, and in common with any early detection programme, there is the problem of dealing with benign disease which clinically or radiologically may mimic breast cancer and in which breast cancer must be excluded and, secondly and more specially to programmes of breast self-examination, there is likely to be an increase in the demand for treatment of symptomatic benign breast disease amongst the population of women who have been specifically asked to look for and report changes in the breast.

Programmes of early detection in breast cancer have reported rates of benign to malignant biopsy as high as 10 : 1, whereas in control populations where no intervention scheme is in operation the ratio of benign to malignant biopsies is generally less than one in the 45–65 year age group. Clearly, therefore, there is a tendency for early detection schemes to produce a marked increase in the number of women undergoing benign (unnecessary) biopsy. In some cases these biopsies are inevitable. If a woman presents with a definite lump in the breast or mammo-

Table 6.1
Reasons for follow-
up of patients within
the self-referral clinic
and the incidence of
carcinoma.

	No. of patients	No. of biopsies	No. with cancer
Clinical abnormality	175	14	2
Mammographic abnormality	139	7	1
Clinical and mammographic abnormality	77	6	1
	391	27	4

graphic signs which are indistinguishable from carcinoma, biopsy is mandatory. There remain grey areas both clinically and on mammographic grounds in which suspicion exists in the mind of the examiner but where there are no definitive signs of malignancy. In an effort to reduce the number of benign (unnecessary) biopsies generated by the self-examination programme, we have, in the self-referral unit, engaged in a policy of careful follow-up rather than immediate biopsy in cases where there is clinical or mammographic doubt. Of the 1295 patients who presented in the first three years of the programme, 391 have been followed up within the unit because of doubtful changes on clinical examination or mammography. The reasons for follow-up within the unit, together with the number of biopsies performed in each group and the yield of cancers found, is shown in Table 6.1, divided into those with clinical abnormality only, those with mammographic abnormality only, and those with both clinical and mammographic abnormalities. A scheme of management for mammographic abnormalities is outlined elsewhere (Chapter 8) and the operation of such a scheme has enabled us to detect the one breast cancer in the group with mammographic abnormalities only while performing only seven biopsies in those 139 patients.

One hundred and seventy-five patients were followed up because of clinical abnormalities present at the time of examination despite the fact that they had a normal mammogram (or at least one which showed benign changes only). The presence of a normal mammogram in these women is reassuring but it must be remembered that mammography may miss up to 10% of all cancers, either because the cancers cannot be seen against the background pattern or because they are in a site which makes visualization on mammography difficult or impossible. The reasons for clinical review are shown in Table 6.2. By far the most common was the finding of lumpy breasts. Any clinician who deals with patients with breast disease will recognize the difficulty which is sometimes encountered in differentiating benign lumpiness from significant pathology. The routine for reviewing these patients has been for the nursing staff to arrange for them to be seen by the clinic doctor in six weeks time or, in premenopausal women, in the week following their next period. If the abnormality is still present at this time and considered to be

Table 6.2
Reasons for clinical review (No. of patients=175) within the self-referral clinic.

134	lumpy breasts
7	skin dimpling or deformity (excluding nipple retraction
12	nipple retraction
15	palpable axillary nodes
2	nipple eczema
9	nipple discharge
1	pain without abnormality
1	resolving abscess
4	no information given

185 (i.e. 10 had combination of two of these)

of possible significance, they are reviewed again at three and six months and in any case where doubt still exists a further mammogram is performed at six months. If, of course, there is any change in the examination findings suggestive of progressive disease, then immediate biopsy is undertaken. By employing this scheme of follow-up, we have been able to detect the two breast cancers amongst the 175 patients presenting with doubtful clinical abnormalities, while performing only 14 biopsies in this group. Although there has been some delay in the diagnosis of these two breast cancers, both were detected at an 'early' stage, both being less than 2 cm in maximum diameter and neither having any node involvement at mastectomy.

By following this defined policy of careful follow-up rather than proceeding to immediate biopsy in doubtful cases, we have managed to keep the benign to malignant biopsy ratio over this period of time down to 0.9 : 1. In addition, the policy of follow-up in the unit allows clear recommendation to be given to both G.P. and patient at the time of discharge. There is no room in any intervention programme for the issuing of ambiguous reports to general practitioners.

Specific complications of a programme of breast self-examination

Management of symptomatic benign disease
If in the course of an early detection programme women are specifically asked to report changes in their breasts or new symptoms, the correct management of symptomatic benign disease is important even when carcinoma can be excluded.

One-third of all patients presenting to the self-referral unit following education have done so complaining of breast pain or discomfort. This is a considerably higher proportion than is seen in the hospital breast clinic and is at least in part due to the education programme itself. Having created a demand for treatment, the correct management of breast pain is important. Most of these women only require reassurance, but in some these symptoms merit treatment in their own right and in these women breast pain can be managed successfully according to the scheme outlined in Chapter 32.

The induction of anxiety

One of the major talking points involved in the use and recommendation of breast self-examination in a mass programme is whether any potential benefits might be outweighed by the induction of anxiety in a large proportion of the population. In addition to the obvious psychological morbidity, this may result in many more patients presenting (sometimes repeatedly) to their general practitioner or hospital clinic without significant pathology.

There is little hard data on this subject but many opinions have been expressed. We have not, in the course of the education programme, specifically sought a history or signs of anxiety amongst the population under study. Certain observations, however, enable us to make some judgement based on our experience from educating this large group of women as to whether significant clinical anxiety is being induced. It would seem likely that such anxiety would, at least to some degree, manifest itself at the self-referral clinic, and indeed a proportion of women have attended the clinic for reassurance concerning long-term symptoms which might otherwise never have presented. The provision of such reassurance is one of the functions of the self-referral clinic.

If anxiety was to prove problematical it would be reflected in two features concerning the use of this clinic. Firstly, one would expect a large number of asymptomatic anxious women to present and this has not happened. Out of an educated population of over 20 000, only 28 women have presented themselves to the clinic while entirely asymptomatic. Secondly, if reassurance could not be provided by the clinic at first attendance and anxiety was rife, one would expect a large number of patients to pay repeated visits to the clinic. In fact, in the first three years that the clinic has been open only 52 patients returned on more than one occasion and, indeed, only six of these on more than two occasions. Of these six, four have had recurrent breast cysts and on each presentation have had significant findings.

This may be an underestimate of the incidence of anxiety since a number of patients with other symptoms, particularly breast pain, might never have presented except for the anxiety induced by education. The problem, however, in this regard is demonstrably small. It should be noted that any screening programme relies on a balance of anxiety as no woman would attend without some degree of concern.

Summary

Whether breast self-examination will save lives remains open to question. It is clear from the results of the Nottingham programme that it can modify the stage at which breast cancer presents.

To be effective, education in breast self-examination must reach as high a proportion of the population as possible.

Attendance at education sessions is increased by personal invitation from the women's own general practitioner. Accurate population registration is essential.

Such a programme generates an increased workload which can be satisfactorily managed in a self-referral unit staffed by appropriately trained nurses and radiographers.

Careful follow-up of doubtful clinical and mammographic abnormalities, as an alternative to immediate biopsy, is safe and reduces the number of unnecessary biopsies by a self-examination programme.

There is no evidence that there is a significant induction of clinically significant anxiety as a result of an early detection programme based on education and breast self-examination.

7 Mammographic Screening

Jillian Haslehurst

In 1976, Marks & Spencer set up a mammographically-based screening programme for its permanent staff. Women over the age of 35 years are invited to attend for clinical examination and mammography every 15 months. To date, 29 024 women have participated in this programme and the overall detection is 5.8 cancers per thousand women screened, which is in line with the results of other centres. Sixty-five per cent of the 169 tumours detected at screening are small (< 2 cm in size, with a mean of 1.23 cm) and 80% are node-negative. This study continues and long-term follow-up will add to the national data base of information on the survival of the women who have been diagnosed as having early breast cancer. The survival curve of the 151 cases followed for a minimum of 18 months is shown in Fig. 7.1. Only 7 have died, one from a cause other than breast cancer.

In addition to the screen-detected cancers, 56 interval cancers have arisen, 12 of which were present in retrospect at the previous screening and have been termed 'missed' cases. Overall, these results are very encouraging but a screening programme carries with it a number of difficulties.

Problems of a mobile screening service
When the service was first organized in 1976, the first problem considered was the provision of facilities in 264 UK stores for competent clinical examination combined with mammography. Three articulated trailer units were equipped with a waiting area, a clinical examination room and a mammography unit. The apparatus installed has generally stood up well to wear and tear over the years. However, when mechanical problems do occur, this entails a great deal of disruption to prebooked appointments, as well as delaying the arrival of the unit at the next store.

To ensure constant quality control of the mammograms, all films are processed daily in London. The radiographers therefore cannot check their films as they are taken and technical faults may not be discovered until the following day when the films are seen. Occasionally, therefore, some X-rays may not be up to the usual standard.

Another problem with a mobile screening service is that both nurses and radiographers spend much of their working lives away from home. This leads to increased staff turnover, meaning

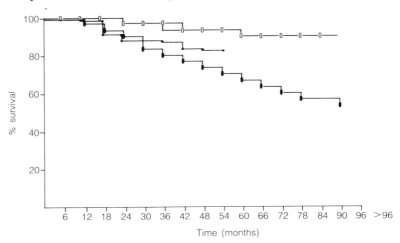

Figure 7.1
Graph of survival of breast cancers detected by mammographic screening (O—O, *n*=149) self-referral after education for self-palpation (·—·, *n*=164) and referral by GP after casual finding of lump (●—●, *n*=772).

that new staff have to be retrained in order to maintain standards.

The recruitment of women to the screening programme
Many screening programmes have a very high acceptance rate during the first year of screening and this subsequently declines as interest wanes or women find that the examination is too uncomfortable to tolerate. It is important to tell women what to expect before their examination so that they are not embarrassed by having to undress to the waist for clinical examination. Also they should be prepared for the slight discomfort experienced by many women during the breast compression required during mammography. These aims have been achieved by the production of a short video film which shows a woman having her history taken, being examined by the nurse, and finally having mammography. This has also been a useful medium to advise women that they should not shave under their arms before screening, as this can cause lymphadenopathy. They are also advised to refrain from using deodorant or talcum powder which can appear as artefacts on the films. These last two points are a continuing problem because when a woman attends for a medical examination she is likely to be particularly scrupulous about personal hygiene.

The acceptance rates of screening at Marks & Spencer indicate the benefit from a company-based programme. The overall acceptance rate has never fallen below 80% (Table 7.1). This can be attributed to prescreening education, peer group pressure, easy availability and finally, and possibly most significantly, the fact that screening is always done during working hours. This experience contrasts with that of two Dutch units, where the acceptance rate over the years after the first examination, fell steadily to less than 50%.

Table 7.1
Acceptance rate by
age group.

Age group	35–39	40–44	45–49	50–54	55–59
Acceptance %	83	90	86	83	80

Problems encountered with distribution of results

Central administration of a nationwide programme brings inevitable delay between the screening examination and availability of results. This delay is about two weeks. For the vast majority of women this does not cause undue alarm, though there is a small minority who do become extremely anxious. Any necessary referral is undertaken by the woman's GP. This can mean delay while the woman waits for appointments, first with her GP and later, her surgeon. This period of waiting causes some anxiety and could probably be reduced by direct liaison between the screening team, local surgeons and local radiologists.

Anxiety regarding breast cancer

The subject of breast cancer is an emotional one for many women. In attending for screening women are accepting the possibility that they may have cancer and that this may be picked up by the methods used. This will inevitably lead to some anxiety but all screening programmes have to generate a certain amount of worry or no one would attend. No woman in our programme has developed an anxiety state warranting psychiatric care.

Another cause for concern in some women is whether or not the compression of the breast tissue during mammography is harmful and these women will need reassurance. A few women are aware that radiation can be potentially harmful and assurance should be given that the radiation dosage used is of an acceptable level. Feig states that there is a risk estimate of 3.5 cancers per million per year per rad, which means that if 1 million women aged 30 years or older had received a minimum dose of 1 rad, there would, after a minimal latent period of 10 years, be an excess incidence of 3.5 cancers each year in the population. Assuming a 50% breast cancer mortality, the hypothetical risk would be one excess death per 2 million women examined. It should be remembered that at age 50 the annual incidence of breast cancer is 1800 cases per million women per year. In addition, the fears of excess leukaemia due to the scatter of radiation to the sternum have not been realized 14 years after the HIP study ceased. The current radiation dosages employed by the Marks & Spencer screening programme are between 0.13 and 0.19 cGy mean dose per breast per film, depending on breast size. Levels are monitored regularly by a physicist at St Bartholomew's Hospital, as control of radiation dosage is mandatory.

Where to refer?
Although referral to specialized breast clinics is ideal, some areas may have inadequate facilities to cope with screening abnormalities. A number of women requiring further mammography, ultrasound or interventive radiological investigations may be referred on to specialized units. If localization of a radiological lesion presents difficulty, one of the team of radiologists in London will undertake this at the request of a surgeon. A flexible fine wire is used to localize the abnormality and the patient returns to her own surgeon for operation the following day.

Benign: Suspicious biopsy ratio
In the 8 years since the inception of the breast screening programme, 29 000 women have participated and 3290 have been advised to see a surgeon. One thousand five hundred and forty-five procedures have been undertaken of which 1376 were benign, and 169 have proved to be carcinomas. The benign:malignant biopsy rate is therefore 8 : 1. This appears to be very high, but this is possibly because cyst aspirations are included in the figures.

Missed and interval cases
No screening programme can hope to be 100% effective and the programme has succeeded in diagnosing 75% of the total number of cancers occurring in the company. However, there have been 44 interval cases in the screened women, and a further 12 missed cases. Missed cases are defined as those in which there was a radiological abnormality visible retrospectively on the X-rays once surgical data is available or if less than a year has elapsed since the previous examination, when there is no radiological abnormality. The interval group are those women who develop a cancer following a previously negative screening examination.

The mean time elapsing from negative mammographic examination to diagnosis of an interval case ranged from 4 to 54 months. The median value fell between 12 and 13 months and this is probably the optimum time interval for a screening programme to be effective. Although not detected by the screening programme, these interval tumours still tend to be quite small (1.7 cm on average) with a node-negative rate of 68%. However, following the diagnosis of an interval breast cancer, the acceptance in that particular store may fall the following year, probably because women begin to doubt the effectiveness of screening.

Radiological abnormalities
Expert radiological assessment is vital to the effectiveness of any screening programme since 99.5% of mammograms taken in an asymptomatic population will be normal. The radiologist is therefore identifying the 0.5% with an abnormality.

Cost
Even in the most economic of programmes, the average cost per

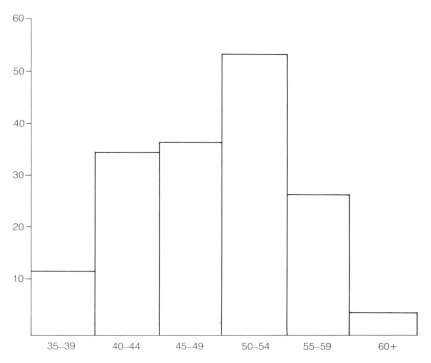

Figure 7.2
Age distribution of
the 169 cancers
detected at screening.

screening examination is about £15. Mammography in the Marks & Spencer scheme costs around £35 per woman, but it should be remembered that most of this cost is incurred because the service is mobile; maintenance of vehicles is expensive, as is subsistence paid to staff. Also, no voluntary help is used at any stage of the programme. Large numbers of examinations must be performed to detect the one case whose prognosis may be favourably affected by early diagnosis. This is true of all detection programmes, but it assumes greater importance when the cost is so high.

Age at which to start screening
The HIP study showed a positive survival benefit in women over the age of 50 years. The Marks & Spencer screening programme has shown that in a working population 50% of the cases of carcinoma are under 50 years. It is important to study the younger group carefully to see if there is a survival benefit in this younger age group. Marks & Spencer begin screening at the age of 35, although only a very few women develop cancer between 35 and 40 years (fig. 7.2).

Age at which to finish screening
The age when screening should cease has not yet been closely scrutinized because currently very few pensioners take part in

the programme. It seems logical to continue screening older women as the disease continues to affect this age group. However, in general, after the age of 65 years enthusiasm for screening declines on the part of the women themselves.

Assessment of effectiveness of screening
A screening programme can be deemed to be effective if fewer women in the screened group die of breast cancer than in the non-screened group. At Marks & Spencer 15–20% of women do not participate in screening. Because of their pension scheme, all deaths are notified to Head Office, so eventually it will be possible to compare the death rates from breast cancer in both the screened and non-screened women.

Conclusion
The past eight years' experience has shown that it is possible to diagnose tumours when they are small and node-negative. By far the best means of doing this is by using mammography since 92% of the screen-detected cancers have positive mammographic findings. It is the only indicator of a problem in over 50% of screen-detected cancers. Six per cent of tumours do not show on mammography.

Many of the problems discussed above can be overcome, providing that the medical and administrative staff are prepared to communicate effectively with each other, and with GPs and surgeons. This demands a high degree of commitment from all staff concerned, both in terms of time and effort.

Further reading
Hutchinson, J. & Tucker, A. (1984) Breast screening results from a healthy working population. *Clin. Oncol.*, *10*, 123–128.

Feig, S. (1979) Epidemiology of radiation related breast cancer. In: *Reduced Dose Mammography*, ed. Logan, W.W. & Muntz, E.P. pp. 10–20. New York: Masson.

8 Mammography

Eric Roebuck

'Mammography is a much more sensitive screening test than clinical examination, may be more cost effective and entails almost negligible radiation hazard.'

In an environment where the art of mammography has developed to a stage when a reputable journal such as the *Lancet* can publish this statement in a leading article, it is not surprising that surgeons will wish to use mammography in the management of patients referred to them with breast problems. Having said that, it is very important to realize that symptomatic patients should not be sent for mammography without a proper prior clinical examination.

Some of the indications for mammography in a general surgical practice are listed in Table 8.1. In the management of breast cancer the contralateral breast should be examined by mammography before definitive treatment is commenced, because about 3% of patients will have contralateral, mammographically detectable but clinically occult, cancer. Prior to treatment by excision/irradiation rather than mastectomy (Chapter 12), a baseline mammogram is taken in order to facilitate early detection of any recurrence and following treatment by excision or radiation mammograms are initially carried out at six-month intervals. Following any treatment for operable primary breast cancer, the development of contralateral cancer may occur (the risk is increased ten times); this certainly justifies regular mammography during follow-up for patients who have a good outlook following the treatment of their first cancer. Patients considered to be at high risk either on grounds of family history or previous biopsy evidence of atypia should have regular mammography (perhaps biennually).

Problems of mammography

To use a mammographic service effectively the difficulties in the techniques involved must be appreciated and overcome and the service must be used appropriately. There are questions which are best answered by mammography and some which mammography cannot answer. To be of acceptable quality, a mammographic service must have a high sensitivity and a high specificity—failure to achieve and maintain these will give rise to difficulties in management.

Mammography is a multistage technical process leading to the demonstration of breast structure on a film. Difficulties arise at each stage in the technical process, which if not eliminated will

Table 8.1		
Indications for mammography in surgical practice.	*Breast cancer*	Contralateral breast Treatment by excision/irradiation
	High risk patients	Strong family history Atypia on previous biopsy
	Benign disease	Clinical doubtful area

result in suboptimal quality or even a failure to demonstrate fine details. Following demonstration, the films are viewed by a radiologist who may make errors of observation or of interpretation. Finally, the opinion resulting from the interpretation has to be communicated to the clinician who, in turn, may not carry out appropriate action. A mammographic service therefore involves radiographic staff and a radiologist and necessitates close liaison between radiologist and the surgeon, together with adequate feedback of pathological findings. More radiographers and radiologists need to be specifically trained in the details of the specialized techniques of mammography and will need to be aware of the objectives of surgical management.

Danger of radiation

Before a mammographic service is instituted, a knowledge of the radiation hazard is essential. There are no data which prove that irradiation of the breast with the radiation doses associated with mammography has a causal relationship with breast cancer.

Extrapolation from experience with much higher doses of more penetrating (higher kv) irradiation than is used in mammography, does suggest there may be a risk assuming a straight line relationship and no threshold. This risk has been calculated (Gravelle et al, 1982) to be in the region of 3.5 cases per 1 000 000 women, per year, per rad of irradiation. Details of the radiation doses associated with mammography are given in Table 8.2 from which the very marked reductions achieved with modern techniques can be appreciated. It is essential that the dose from mammography is minimized by good technique and by avoiding unnecessary examinations. In this respect efforts should be directed towards determining management on the basis of the first mammogram without resorting to repeat examinations unless this is absolutely essential.

Table 8.2		
Radiation dose to the mid breast for single exposures with various techniques.	*Technique*	*Mid-breast dose* (rads)
	Non-screen films	0.8–1.2
	Film/screen combinations	
	Early 1970s	0.10
	Late 1970s	0.05
	Early 1980s	0.02

Regular mammography should be avoided in young (< 35 years of age) non-symptomatic women, but there is no reason to avoid a single mammogram in the symptomatic women of that age if clinical examination indicates that this would be of benefit.

Technical difficulties
A mammographic image must have excellent resolution and good contrast between adjacent structures. To obtain this result a radiation beam with a narrow energy spectrum, in the 25–30 kV range, must be matched to an appropriate receptor system. This is usually a film and intensifying screen combination, but in some centres a Xeroradiographic technique is preferred. Accurate positioning of the patient is mandatory, and good compression is essential to reduce image unsharpness. Degradation of the final image by scattered radiation can be reduced by accurate collimation and the use of an anti-scatter grid.

With a young patient with dysplasia, mammographic details of pathological significance may be hidden amongst non-significant and normal, but dense, shadowing. However, with improvement in techniques, mammography is becoming more accurate even in this age group. For example in a series reported by Moskowitz et al (1977), 67% of the in-situ and < 0.5 cm diameter cancers in women aged 35–44 years were detected by mammography alone.

The size of the patient's breasts also has a bearing on mammographic quality—the extremely large breast usually contains a large proportion of fat and is less of a problem than the unusually small. In these cases the difficulties encountered in positioning the breast on the X-ray film and in applying adequate compression can easily result in incomplete demonstration. In addition in these circumstances the technique of mammography can be painful.

Difficulties of observation
In order to achieve a high sensitivity in a mammographic service it is essential to eliminate perceptual errors. If viewing conditions are suboptimal, many mammographic abnormalities will not be observed. Viewing boxes should be provided with screens to cut out surrounding glare, and a small bright light source should be available together with a large magnifying lens. However, even with these facilities some errors of observation will occur.

In a review of the cancers missed in four high quality American breast cancer detection centres, 29% of the missed lesions were obvious oversights on the part of the original examiner (Martin et al, 1979). In attempts to minimize this group of patients, a double reading technique has been proved to be successful in several centres. The relatively less experienced film readers are better in the detection of mass lesions and clusters of calcifications (sensitivity) than in the accurate diagnosis of cancer (specificity). This indicates that although double reading assists in observation, experience assumes a greater importance when it comes to interpretation.

One common cause of perceptive errors which is more likely to occur with the relatively inexperienced is the obsession with an obvious abnormality, and the overlooking of coexistent more subtle signs of equal or greater pathological significance. This may account for the wide spectrum of reported rates of simultaneous contralateral cancers which varies from 0.3% up to 3.6%.

Difficulties in interpretation

1 *Mass lesions*
The feature of greatest significance to be identified in the differentiation of benign from malignant mass lesions is the interface between the lesion and the surrounding breast parenchyma—a clearly identified margin (Fig. 8.1), possibly with a halo of fat, signifying benignity, whereas a lack of

Figure 8.1
Benign lesion (arrowed) in dysplastic breast, showing halo of fat.

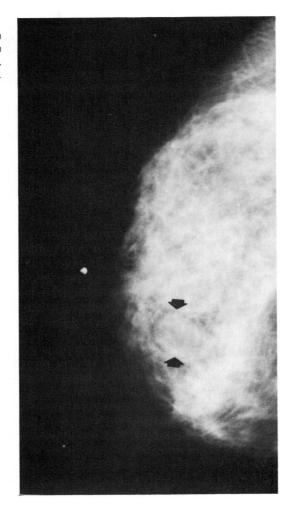

Figure 8.2
Ultrasound showing
cysts: enhancement
behind one cyst is
well shown. (Figure
kindly provided by
Dr Adrian Manhire,
Nottingham City
Hospital.)

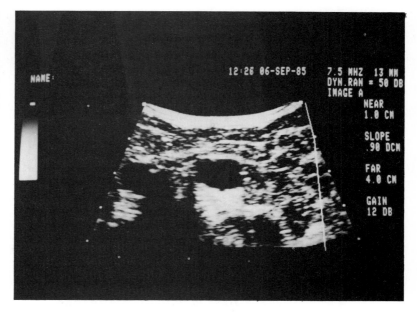

definition of all or of a segment of the margin raises the
probability of malignancy.

Difficulties in delineation of the margin arise if the surrounding breast parenchyma is dense or if the radiographic technique has been less than perfect. In these cases, reliance must
be placed on other features or, alternatively, in the use of
additional modalities: ultrasound (Fig. 8.2) will accurately
differentiate cystic from solid lesions down to a diameter of 0.5
cm and will in many cases differentiate benign solid lesions
from malignant, provided the diameter of the lesion is greater
than about 1 cm. The position of the mass lesion within a breast
relative to the visible glandular tissue is of importance. Even a
well-defined lesion which lies outside the gland tissue should
be regarded as likely to be malignant.

2 *Cysts*

Breast cysts are extremely common. Careful scrutiny of a
mammogram will reveal several and often numerous 2–3 cm
diameter cysts in about 50% of breasts of women in their
forties. If a cyst recurs several times in the same position, or,
very unusually, the aspirate of a cyst contains fresh blood, then
a pneumocystogram may be performed (Fig. 8.3). In the latter
situation, the needle should be left in situ at the end of the
aspiration and a volume of air equal to that of the aspirate
injected. A mammogram film taken within one hour identifies
or excludes the presence of an intracystic lesion.

Figure 8.3
Pneumocystogram
showing intracystic
lesion.

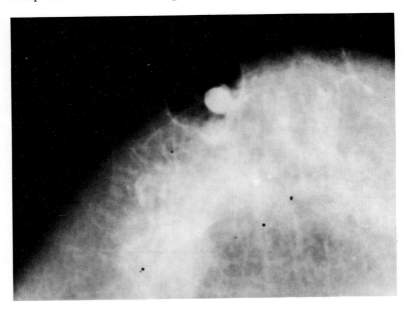

Figure 8.3
Pneumocystogram showing intracystic lesion.

3 *Microcalcification*

Microcalcification is of the utmost importance in the identification of malignancy and is the most common sign in in-situ carcinomas. If microcalcifications are dense for their size, or of irregular shapes (particularly if rod-like or branching calcifications are present), or if they are arranged in rows or clusters, then malignancy should be suspected. However, sclerosing adenosis can produce calcification which is of identical appearance to that associated with malignancy. This difficulty is lessened if the calcifications lie in several regions within the breast, and particularly if the changes are bilateral, when sclerosing adenosis is more likely. Even then, the possibility of multifocal in-situ cancer must be considered, and in these cases a repeat examination after an interval of six months is necessary in order to identify the presence of a progressive lesion.

In addition to sclerosing adenosis, calcifications indistinguishable from those associated with malignancy can be present due to the more severe states of ductal epitheliosis and hyperplasia.

4 *Stellate lesions*

The classical appearances of a small carcinoma (Fig. 8.5), consisting of a mass with spicules extending into the surrounding parenchyma, can be mimicked by a radial scar (Figs 8.4, 8.5). On occasion, a radiolucent centre will suggest the latter diagnosis, as may the presence of very thin spicules. Traumatic

Figure 8.4
Radial scar.

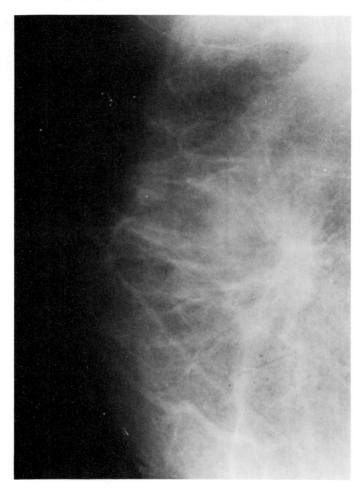

fat necrosis and, rarely, myxoid degeneration of a fibroadenoma can also present a scirrhous carcinoma-like appearance.

Radiologist's
recommendations
Inevitably, some benign lesions will be referred for biopsy on
mammographic grounds, particularly sclerosing adenosis and
epitheliosis, but with high quality radiological interpretation
the proportion can be less than 2:1.

Having made his observations and interpretations, a radiologist should then be in a position to quantify his degree of
confidence in his mammographic diagnosis. Unless this is done, a
large number of benign abnormalities will be referred for biopsy.
If a lesion is identified it is recommended that the degree of
confidence in its nature be expressed on a five-point scale ranging
from definitely malignant, through probably malignant,

Figure 8.5
Carcinoma plus radial
scar.

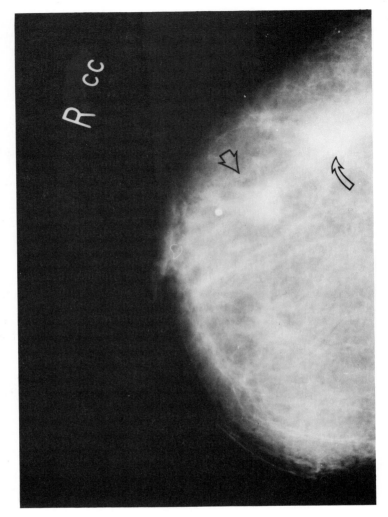

indeterminate, probably benign to definitely benign. This requires considerable discipline on the part of the radiologist.

The five points on the malignant to benign scale each imply a specific management recommendation (Table 8.3).
Follow-up is by a predetermined scheme, designed to identify cancers as early as possible and over a period sufficiently long to ensure that any progression of mammographic signs will become apparent. By undertaking a clinical examination at 6 and 12 weeks in the follow-up period, with a repeat mammogram and clinical examination at six months, it is highly unlikely that any cancers will be missed. Indeed, in our population monitoring study no missed cancers have arisen once this scheme was adopted.

Table 8.3
Relationship between
radiologist's opinion
and management
recommendation.

Radiologist's opinion	Management recommendation
Malignant	Biopsy
Probably malignant	Biopsy
Indeterminate	Follow-up
Probably benign	Follow-up
Benign	Discharge

Clearly a clinical assessment of the patient may modify the mammographic assessment in the determination of management. If biopsy is indicated on either mammographic or clinical grounds, then biopsy should not be delayed by normal findings in the other modality.

Communication with the surgeon

A formalized scheme, such as suggested above, eliminates a major difficulty which arises in the communication between radiologist and clinicians when it is often difficult to express the subtlety of the significance of clinical signs observed in a mammogram. It is necessary to ensure that the radiologist is part of a team rather than, as in so many centres at present, merely issuing reports in isolation.

Conclusion

For a mammographic service to be of value in the management of breast disease, it is essential to ensure that radiographic expertise is such that the mammographic images are of the highest quality. Unless radiologists take a special interest in mammography, they will be incapable of ensuring that the radiographic quality remains high and it is likely that they will generate reports which will result in an unduly high rate of benign biopsies. It is of importance that any radiologist participating in mammography should be specifically trained in this specialized area. Without close liaison between radiologist and surgeon, the dangers of a mammographic service are such that patients and surgeons will inevitably be falsely reassured or pushed into unnecessary operative procedures. Mammography in the symptomatic patient should never be undertaken without a competent prior clinical examination and we do not recommend an open mammography service for GPs in investigations of the symptomatic patient.

References and Further reading

Gravelle, H.S.E., Simpson, P.R. & Chamberlain, J. (1982) Breast cancer screening and health service costs. *J. Health Econ.*, *1*, 185–207.

Martin, J.E., Moskowitz, M. & Milbrath, J.R. (1979) Breast cancer missed by mammography. *Am. J. Roentgenol.*, *132*, 737–739.

Moskowitz, M., Gartside, P., Gardella, L., De Groot, I. & Guenther, D.

(1977) The breast screening controversy: a perspective. *Am. J. Roentgenol., 129,* 537–547.

Price, J.L. & Gibbs, N.M. (1978) The relationship between microcalcification and in situ carcinomas of the breast. *Clin. Radiol., 29,* 447–452.

Roebuck, E.J. (1983) *Techniques in Diagnostic Radiology,* ed. Whitehouse, G.H. & Worthington, B.S. pp. 314–324. Oxford: Blackwell Scientific Publications.

Thomas, B.A., Price, J.L. & Bolter, P.S. (1983) The Guildford Breast Screening Project. *Clin. Oncol., 9,* 121–129.

Venet, L., Strax, P., Venet, W. & Shapiro, S. (1972) Adequacies and inadequacies of breast examinations by physicians in mass screening. *Cancer, 29,* 1546–1551.

9 The Treatment of Primary Breast Cancer

Roger Blamey

For some 70 years after the time of Halsted, the accepted treatment of primary breast cancer was wide excision linked to an extensive dissection of the draining nodes. To this was often added radiotherapy, both to flaps and to nodes. The side-effects of this extensive treatment to the local disease are recounted in Chapter 10.

Several lines of approach led to a change in the therapy for primary disease. A number of clinical trials were carried out using progressively less radical treatments to reach the present regimen. Now many surgeons would consider simple mastectomy, without an attack on the draining nodes, as satisfactory treatment for the primary growth (Fig. 9.1). Alongside the trials came long-term follow-up studies, such as that of Brinkley and Haybittle (1975) (Fig. 9.2), which demonstrated that despite wide removal of the primary growth and therapy to the draining nodes, the majority of patients with even Stage I and II breast cancer eventually died of their disease. Clearly, most patients already have distant metastases spread through the blood stream at the time of diagnosis, rather than temporarily arrested in the draining nodes. At the same time as this change in medical thinking, the patients themselves have come to understand far more about breast cancer and choose therapies which are both less extensive and give a better cosmetic appearance.

Thus in Nottingham we have moved towards breast conservation, through reconstruction by subcutaneous mastectomy to excision of the primary tumour followed by high dose irradiation. The results and side-effects are described in Chapters 11 and 12. The early result of the recent trial conducted in the USA by the NSABP has shown that breast conservation using local excision of the tumour plus irradiation does not worsen survival in comparison with mastectomy. However, excision without subsequent irradiation is followed by a very high incidence of local recurrence.

Why, then, do we not offer treatment by excision/irradiation to all patients with primary breast cancer? The first objective before a new treatment is accepted is that survival must be of the same order as previous treatments, the second is that subsequent uncontrolled local recurrence must not be a problem. Some of our patients have developed uncontrolled local recurrence: these

Figure 9.1
Cancer Research
Campaign Trial:
WP=patients
treated by simple
mastectomy and
'watched';
DXT=patients
treated by simple
mastectomy with
prophylactic irra-
diation of flaps and
node areas. Sur-
vival to 14 years is
seen to be indepen-
dent of which treat-
ment was used.
(Figure kindly pro-
vided by Professor
Michael Baum.)

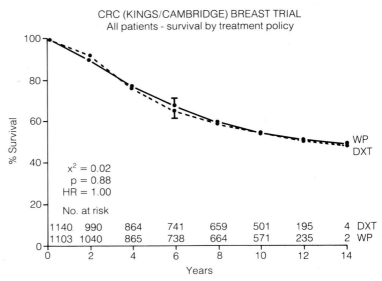

Figure 9.1 Cancer Research Campaign Trial: WP=patients treated by simple mastectomy and 'watched'; DXT=patients treated by simple mastectomy with prophylactic irradiation of flaps and node areas. Survival to 14 years is seen to be independent of which treatment was used. (Figure kindly provided by Professor Michael Baum.)

came from the group with particularly aggressive tumours (see Chapter 12). Local recurrence in this group is a problem even after mastectomy but failure of subsequent local control may not be as common. The other group who appear at this early stage to be possibly unsuitable for treatment by excision/irradiation are those patients with carcinoma-in-situ (Chapter 12) and in Nottingham we are at present not offering this treatment for carcinoma-in-situ.

Because we believe that breast conservation or reconstruction is likely to diminish depressive states and generally to improve the quality of life for breast cancer patients, our policy is to offer such treatments. The diagnosis made (Chapter 1) the surgeon, counselling sister, patient and usually her husband discuss the illness and the methods of treating the primary disease. The patient is told that the simplest method of treatment, involving only one operation, is simple mastectomy. Subcutaneous mastectomy, its complications and cosmetic results are described: contrasted with the other two choices, this operation is falling out of favour. Excision/irradiation is described as a procedure which does not carry a guarantee of long-term results, a procedure which carries approximately a 10% chance of local recurrence requiring mastectomy, and a procedure which requires rigorous follow-up including mammography and, possibly, frequent Trucut biopsy: all this is in addition to the six weeks of irradiation treatment.

Given the alternatives set out in this way, young women overwhelmingly choose breast conservation and the great majority of women over 60 opt for simple mastectomy.

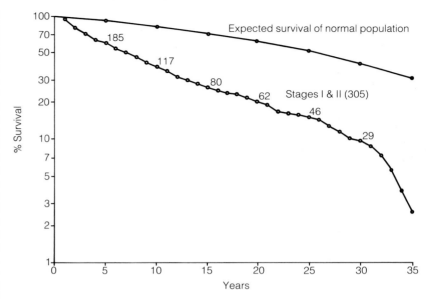

Figure 9.2
Survival of 305 cases of Stage I and II primary breast cancer followed over 35 years, compared with actuarial survival of the population. Although numbers at risk are small at the end of the curve there is evidence of a higher death rate in the cancer group even at 30–35 years: death directly from breast cancer still contributes to this death rate. (Figure kindly provided by Dr. John Haybittle.)

The patient discusses the impending operation with the counselling sister. It has been found that the period after treatment and discharge from hospital is the time of maximum depression and anxiety. In an effort to combat this, the breast counselling volunteers (all of whom have undergone treatment for primary breast cancer) visit the patient at home. The patient regularly attends a follow-up clinic; the fitter of protheses is another member of the team regularly available in the clinic for patients to consult.

Clinic follow-up is arranged three-monthly for the first 24 months (36 months for excision/irradiation) and then six-monthly.

The facilities of counselling, the reassurance of follow-up investigation, availability of protheses and swimwear, etc., attendance of a psychiatrist when required (Chapter 15), are all features of the specialist breast clinic. Such an arrangement is even more necessary in secondary breast disease and for procedures connected with breast cancer screening. It is to be hoped that surgeons in the future will let personal pride be subservient to the requirement for one surgeon in each centre to specialize in breast disease to some extent in order to establish a service with these facilities, to the assured benefit of the unfortunate patients.

Patients with locally advanced primary cancer are not treated in this way (see Chapter 14) and patients over the age of 70 years may be better managed by endocrine treatment as the first approach (Preece, 1985): the comparison between tamoxifen and mastectomy as the first line of treatment in the over-seventies is the subject of a clinical trial in Nottingham.

Further reading

Brinkley, D. & Haybittle, J.L. (1975) The curability of breast cancer. *Lancet, ii*, 95–97.

Cancer Research Campaign Working Party (1980) Cancer Research Campaign (King's/Cambridge) Trial for early breast cancer. A detailed update at the tenth year. *Lancet, ii*, 55–60.

Fisher, B., Bauer, M., Margolese, R. et al (1985) Five-year results of a randomized clinical trial comparing total mastectomy and segmental mastectomy with or without radiation in the treatment of breast cancer. *New Eng. J. Med., 312*, 665–673.

Halsted, W. (1898) A clinical and histological study of certain adeno-carcinomata of the breast. *J. Am. Surg. Ass., 15*, 114–181.

Preece, P.E. (1985) Treatment of primary breast cancer in women over 70 years of age. In: *Seminar: Breast Cancer*, ed. Blamey, R.W. pp. 31–33. London: Update Publications.

10 Mastectomy and Radiotherapy

John Simpson

This chapter will consider the use of simple (or in the USA 'total') mastectomy and radiotherapy which is regarded as being generally safe and well tolerated and is one of the most commonly used forms of primary therapy. It will also discuss the problems and complications associated with the use of these treatments.

Removal of the whole breast has been used for the treatment of breast cancer for at least 300 years. Severinus, in the seventeenth century, and Syme and Paget, in the nineteenth century, are all reported to have performed this operation, but its use was then generally restricted to locally advanced disease. Halsted (1894) is credited with having established radical mastectomy as a treatment for breast cancer, and providing a scientific rationale for its use. He reported greatly improved local control rates and a ten year survival of approximately 12% (Lewis and Reinhoff, 1932). Due to Halsted's work, radical mastectomy became the standard primary therapy for the first 70 years of this century.

Radiotherapy was first used for the treatment of breast cancer in the early 1900s but its widespread use was delayed until the 1940s (Del Regato, 1971). Initially, it was used after radical mastectomy but later, largely through the efforts of McWhirter (1948), simple mastectomy and radiotherapy became accepted as a reasonable alternative to the Halsted operation. By 1969, this was the single most commonly used form of primary therapy in Britain for 'early' breast cancer (Breast Cancer Symposium, 1969). This was the conclusion of a survey in which Fellows of the Association of Surgeons of Great Britain were asked about their views on management of breast cancer. It has remained a widely practised form of management although the use of postoperative radiotherapy has undoubtedly become more selective. In the United States total mastectomy and radiotherapy has never achieved the same level of acceptance and in 1972, radical mastectomy was still the most widely used operation (Vana et al, 1981). Since then, the Halsted operation has steadily been replaced by modified radical mastectomy and in 1980 the N.I.H. Consensus Development Conference (Moxley et al, 1980) designated total mastectomy and axillary dissection as 'the current standard treatment'.

The decision by many British surgeons to change from radical mastectomy to simple mastectomy was based on the desire to reduce treatment morbidity without compromising the results of treatment. Only limited comparative data on morbidity are available (Roberts et al, 1972), so it is hard to judge the success of the change in these terms.

In considering the various treatment options for the primary treatment of breast cancer, it is important to be aware of the differences that may exist between these options, in terms of survival rates, local recurrence rates, and factors influencing quality of life. Quality of life assessment is a comparatively recent addition to treatment evaluation and is only included in a small minority of contemporary studies. Much has been written about surgical morbidity but comparatively few data have come from randomized studies. This means that comparative rates for the incidence of particular complications are not readily available.

The results of controlled trials which compare the various surgical and radiotherapy options are summarized in Table 10.1. It can be seen that the various treatment options all give comparable prospects of survival. There is the expected consistent trend of local recurrence rates being lower when radiotherapy or more radical surgery is used. Simple mastectomy and radiotherapy appears to be at least comparable with the other options for both survival and local recurrence rates. The remainder of this chapter will be devoted to complications associated with this method of primary therapy.

Complications of treatment
Simple mastectomy and postoperative radiotherapy is generally safe and well tolerated form of therapy for localized breast cancer. Serious complications are rare and deaths, during the hospital admission, are extremely rare.

Non-fatal complications can occur during the operation, in the early postoperative period, or later. Complications will be discussed, separately, for these three time periods. Although this chapter is primarily devoted to simple mastectomy and radiotherapy, some complications of other forms of mastectomy will be considered briefly. If axillary dissection or sampling is performed as part of the mastectomy operation, some of the complications associated with radical mastectomy may be experienced.

Operative complications   Excessive blood loss leading to hypovolaemia and shock is hopefully rare, and can only result from either a major vessel injury or very prolonged ooze from multiple sites. Blood loss requiring transfusion is also uncommon and should occur in no more than 15–20% of patients. Suitable use of diathermy coagulation and careful control of the perforating branches of the internal mammary vessels should ensure that the blood loss will be no more than 150–500 ml.

1 *Nerve and blood vessel injuries*
Mastectomy should not be associated with any significant risk

Table 10.1 Results of controlled trials involving mastectomy.

Trial	Reference	Number of patients	Primary therapy used	Results	
				Survival	*Local recurrence*
International Multicentre	Lacour, J. et al (1983)	1453	Radical mastectomy vs Extended radical mastectomy	No difference at 10 years	Decreased with extended operation
Manchester	Easson, E.C. (1969)	1461	Radical mastectomy vs Radical mastectomy + radiotherapy	No difference at 10 years	Decreased with radiotherapy
Edinburgh	Langlands, A.O. et al (1980)	498	Radical mastectomy vs Simple mastectomy + radiotherapy	Advantage to radical mastectomy ($P=.05$) at 12 years	Decreased with radical mastectomy
Cancer Research Campaign (CRC)	CRC Working Party (1980)	2243	Simple mastectomy + radiotherapy vs Simple mastectomy + watch policy	No difference at 8 years	Decreased with radiotherapy
NSABP B-04	Fisher, B. et al (1980)	1765	Radical mastectomy vs Total mastectomy + radiotherapy (node-positive clinically)	No difference	No difference
			Radical mastectomy vs Total mastectomy + radiotherapy vs Total mastectomy (node-negative clinically)	No difference	Small increase in local + regional recurrence with total mastectomy

of nerve injury and with only minor sensory change over the skin flaps. Any form of axillary dissection will usually lead to division of the intercostobrachial nerve with associated axillary and upper arm numbness. This loss of sensation is permanent, but is rarely a cause of concern to the patient after the first few weeks. She should be warned preoperatively about the expected sensory changes. This nerve can be identified and preserved at operation, but at the expense of making axillary dissection more difficult. The long thoracic nerve, supplying serratus anterior, and the thoracodorsal nerve, supplying latissimus dorsi, are both prone to surgical injury during axillary exploration. Rates for nerve injury as high as 4.9% have been reported by Say and Donegan (1974). Long thoracic nerve injury leads to the unsightly 'winged scapula' deformity, whereas thoracodorsal nerve division produces only mild weakness of shoulder abduction. In a planned anatomical axillary dissection both nerves are identified and their preservation is a surgical routine. In 'sampling' procedures the risk of straying anatomically may possibly be greater although this is not the experience in Nottingham where only a single node is removed from each area (triple node biopsy).

Major vessel injuries are restricted to very occasional damage to the axillary vein. The axillary artery lies above and behind the vein and should be safe from even a moderately disorientated surgeon.

2 *Wound closure and skin flap problems*

One of the more difficult technical aspects of mastectomy is planning the excision of skin so that (a) an adequate margin of skin is removed from the region of the tumour, (b) wound closure is possible without tension, and (c) the resulting wound is cosmetically acceptable. The planning is aided considerably by the use of a marking pen to identify the boundaries of the tumour and the proposed lines of excision of the skin elipse. Usually skin closure without tension is readily achieved but occasionally a split-skin graft is required.

Skin flap necrosis is a common problem and can lead to wound infection and delayed healing. It results from an inadequate blood supply to the flap, which in turn can be caused by rough tissue-handling and excessive tension in wound closure. Thick skin flaps have been shown to lead to a lower incidence of wound problems than thin flaps, and no disadvantage in terms of tumour recurrence (Krohn et al, 1982). Thick skin flaps enable buried subcutaneous sutures to be used to approximate the flaps, and cosmetically-acceptable skin closure can then be achieved with a continuous monofilament subcuticular suture. This type of closure avoids the cross-hatching associated with the use of conventional interrupted sutures.

'Button-holing' of the skin flaps is hopefully uncommon and is more an injury to surgical pride than a real complication. Inevitably there is a risk of skin infarction around the 'button-hole', but unless an area of skin with impaired blood supply is created around the hole, infarction is unlikely. This complication can be avoided by using skin hooks to lift the skin edges vertically while the flaps are being cut.

3 *Pneumothorax*

This is a rare complication of radical mastectomy and an even rarer one of simple mastectomy. In Nottingham a clinical pneumothorax has occurred on three occasions out of some 1300 procedures involving removal of an internal mammary node during triple node biopsy.

At triple node biopsy there has also been one haemothorax requiring postoperative treatment.

Early postoperative complications

A number of problems are experienced between the time of mastectomy and the start of radiotherapy, a period of usually between three and six weeks.

1 *Wound infection*

This is a problem in a significant proportion of patients with rates of about 8% being reported. In Beatty's series (1983) there was a clear relationship between the type of preliminary biopsy performed and the prospects of infection. When only needle biopsy was performed the infection rate was 3.2% and, by contrast, a rate of 23% was found when open biopsy was performed four to seven days before mastectomy. A one-step open biopsy to mastectomy resulted in a rate of 5.3%. All wound infections in this series were due to either *Staphylococcus aureus* or a beta-haemolytic *Streptococcus*. Contamination of the mastectomy wound can take place in the operating theatre or when drains or dressings are being attended to. The unblocking of suction drains may lead to wound infection if attention to sterile technique is not meticulously followed. Host factors which predispose to wound infection include: old age, obesity, diabetes mellitus and poor nutritional status, all of which are fairly common in women with breast cancer. Wound haematomas or seromas provide an excellent culture medium for organisms as does dead or infarcted tissue in the wound. It seems appropriate to consider seriously the use of short course prophylactic antibiotics in, at least, older patients who have had a previous open biopsy. In other types of surgery, particularly involving the gastrointestinal tract, prophylactic antibiotics have an established role in lowering infection rates in high risk patients. Wound infection is a significant complication in terms of immediate morbidity and delayed convalescence, but most importantly in terms of the later development of arm lymphoedema. This aspect of the morbidity of mastectomy wound infection is generally not appreciated by nursing and junior medical staff.

2 *Seroma*
Serous fluid collects to some extent after every mastectomy. The operation creates dead space beneath the skin flaps and in the axilla and in this space lymph and blood collect in the early postoperative period. The nature of the operation ensures that many lymphatics and small blood vessels are divided and seepage will take place from these vessels. Suction drainage is used routinely to remove this fluid collection and to prevent the accumulation of sufficient fluid to cause a palpable swelling or pain. The drainage system is left in place until the drainage for a 24 hour period is down to less than 25 ml. This may occur within three to four days or take as long as three weeks. The development of a seroma (a symptomatic swelling on the medial wall of the axilla) represents either a failure of the drainage system or may occur after the drains have been removed. Say and Donegan (1974) report that it occurs in 30% of total mastectomies and 40% of radical mastectomies. It is therefore a common problem which the patient should be warned about in the very early postoperative period. It can readily be treated by aspiration although this procedure may need to be repeated a number of times.

Suggested methods of preventing seroma formation include closure of the wound dead space by sutures, but most surgeons see seroma as a fairly minor problem and do not use this technique. It does, however, increase the chances of other complications including flap necrosis, delayed wound healing and early lymphoedema and probably warrants being taken more seriously than it is at present.

3 *Scar problems*
Wound infection and skin flap necrosis inevitably lead to more scar tissue deposition in the healing mastectomy wound. The wound will, therefore, both look and feel less satisfactory. Measures to avoid these problems have already been discussed. The direction of the scar influences its eventual appearance with horizontal scars being more generally acceptable to the patients than either oblique or vertical ones. 'Dog-ears' may occur at either end of the mastectomy wound if care is not taken to avoid this problem. Suitable planning of the excision with wide angles being produced at either end make a 'dog-ear' unlikely. In very obese patients some degree of 'dog-ear' at the axillary end of the wound is inevitable. It is sometimes necessary to revise the wound ends either during wound

closure or by a small local anaesthetic procedure performed some time later.

4 *Shoulder stiffness*
Virtually every woman will experience some difficulties in achieving a full range of shoulder movements after mastectomy. Early mobilization with the help of a physiotherapist should ensure that a full range of movements is acquired well within the first postoperative month. This early mobilization may increase the rate of production of lymphatic fluid in the wound but return of shoulder function is judged by most surgeons to be of greater importance. Long-term stiffness is an occasional complication which usually results from inadequate early efforts to regain a full range of movements. Mobilization can begin gently on the first day after mastectomy and the woman should leave hospital with an exercise programme to perform at home.

5 *Early lymphoedema*
Occasionally, arm swelling may be apparent within a few days of surgery but essentially lymphoedema is a late complication. It will be considered in detail in the next section.

Late complications
Included in this group are the late complications of surgery and those complications caused by radiotherapy.

1 *Lymphoedema* (Fig. 10.1)
Increase in girth of the arm on the side of the mastectomy is a common and important problem. It is rarely severe, but when it is, it can cause considerable physical handicap and great distress. The true incidence of lymphoedema is hard to assess because its recognition is so dependent on how it is defined. A usual requirement is for there to be a difference of at least 2 cm in the diameter of the two arms 15 cm below the coracoid process. Incidence figures as low as 2.7% and as high as 72% have been reported. The incidence varies with the type of surgery performed and is more common after radical mastectomy than after total mastectomy alone. Say and Donegan report rates of 31% for radical mastectomy and 9% for simple mastectomy.

The addition of radiation to surgery increases the incidence, with the highest rates resulting from radical surgery followed by radiotherapy. The time of onset of lymphoedema varies from the first one to two weeks postoperatively up to several years later. The highest frequency is found two to four months after surgery with some reduction in incidence after this time (Brismar and Ljungdahl, 1983).

The primary aetiology of the condition is surgical interruption of the lymphatic pathways in the axilla. It is clear that if a

Figure 10.1
Lymph oedema due
to carcinomatous
infiltration at the base
of the neck.

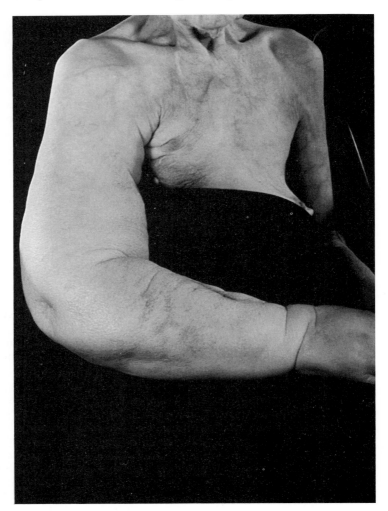

Figure 10.1 Lymph oedema due to carcinomatous infiltration at the base of the neck.

complete axillary dissection is performed, the disturbance of lymphatic anatomy will be greater. It is thought that some restoration of continuity of the lymphatic channels occurs within a few months of surgery due to the growth of new lymph vessels. Radiotherapy appears to prevent and retard this process and causes compression of the remaining vessels due to the development of interstitial fibrosis. Venous obstruction is not thought to be an important factor in the development of lymphoedema.

Infection is an important predisposing factor to the condition. This can be in the form of a mastectomy wound infection or a cellulitis of the arm. Both these conditions are to some extent preventable, a good example being a drip-site infection which leads to cellulitis and lymphoedema. Britton and Nelson (1962) report that 53% of patients with lymphoedema have had an episode of cellulitis at some time.

Lymphoedema is a condition in which prevention is much more successful than attempts to cure the established condition. It is worthwhile to brief nursing and junior medical staff on the importance of treating the upper limb on the side of the mastectomy with great care. Drips, venepuncture and blood pressure measurements on that side should be avoided. The patient should be given, before discharge from hospital, a set of written instructions which will help her to avoid this complication.

The prompt treatment of a developing cellulitis with antibiotics, active against both staphylococci and streptococci, is vital. The limb should be elevated and hospital admission is required for any established infection. In the early postoperative period the intermittent use of a sling together with the use of an elastic sleeve is generally effective in controlling minor degrees of swelling. For longstanding or severe oedema, use of an intermittent mechanical compression device such as the Flowtron may enable the swelling of the arm to be kept to a reasonable level, and allow normal function to take place. Lymphoedema tends to become hard and non-compressible when it has been present for a number of years. When this stage has been reached, surgical treatment is all that can be attempted. Various types of surgery have been tried for this condition including lymphaticovenous shunting, anastomosis of deep and superficial lymphatics, the use of a buried dermal flap, and radical excision of all oedematous tissue with split-skin grafting. None of these methods has become clearly established as the surgical answer to this problem.

A dire complication of longstanding severe lymphoedema is lymphangiosarcoma of the limb (Stewart–Treves syndrome). This is said to occur between one and 27 years after mastectomy in about 10% of all women with severe lymphoedema, and is usually fatal.

2 *Nerve entrapment*
This condition also involving the upper limb is an unpleasant syndrome consisting of paraesthesia, weakness and arm pain. It is caused by compression of nerves in the region of the brachial plexus or the carpal tunnel. It is accompanied by lymphoedema in at least 50% of patients. It must be distinguished from the effects of tumour recurrence and from radiation damage to the brachial plexus. CT scanning and electromyography are useful in excluding recurrent disease and in localizing the site of entrapment. Surgical release is indicated if the carpal tunnel is the site of the entrapment.

3 *Radiation effects*
These are generally mild and transient or more long-term but of limited consequence to the patient. There are, however, a number of major complications recorded, including deaths directly attributable to the effects of radiotherapy, radiation-induced cardiomyopathies and a brain abscess in a patient with persistent leukopaenia.

Radiotherapy for breast cancer causes a number of early side-effects including erythema, desquamation and pigmentation of the skin, and localized pneumonitis. Clinically detectable pneumonitis occurs in about 10% of patients, six to 12 weeks after radiotherapy. The clinical condition resolves, but is followed after six to 12 months by radiologically detectable pulmonary fibrosis. Osteonecrosis of the clavicle, scapula or ribs is a painful complication occurring in 22% of patients treated by radiotherapy (Langlands et al, 1977). A rare but important late complication is an unusual form of peripheral vascular disease which affects irradiated arteries such as the axillary artery.

4 *Malignant complications of radiotherapy*
Non-mammary malignant tumours can develop in the irradiated field as a late complication of radiotherapy. These tumours have usually been reported between ten and 20 years after irradiation (Ferguson et al, 1984). Second tumours developing in this way include oesophageal carcinoma, squamous carcinoma of the skin, and a variety of sarcomas. With the exception of lymphangiosarcoma, which is said to occur in 0.5% of all women treated for breast cancer, the sarcomas are all very rare.

5 *Psychosocial morbidity*
Perhaps the most important complication of mastectomy is the cost in emotional and social terms. There is clear evidence of considerable psychosocial morbidity after mastectomy (Morris, 1979) but it is difficult to separate the effects of breast loss from the impact of a diagnosis of breast cancer. Twenty-five per cent of patients experience anxiety or depression, or both, in the first year after mastectomy and 46% experience sexual difficulties (Maguire et al, 1978). These figures are significantly higher than in a control population with benign breast disease. Important questions arise about the impact of breast-conserving surgery and breast reconstruction on this type of morbidity. It is also interesting to speculate on whether or not the knowledge that mastectomy could be avoided would lead to earlier presentation of women with breast cancer. These questions can be answered by carefully designed studies.

Summary
Simple mastectomy, with or without postoperative radiotherapy,

has become the standard primary therapy for 'early' breast cancer in many British centres.

The psychosocial morbidity of mastectomy is considerable but can be lessened by counselling and patient support. Other forms of treatment morbidity are generally non-severe with major complications being rare. Lymphoedema of the arm is perhaps the most troublesome common complication and is one that is difficult to treat when established. It is, however, usually preventable by careful avoidance of wound and arm infections. Radiation-induced complications are generally transient and non-severe. Major radiation morbidity is almost always avoidable by careful therapy, planning and delivery.

Simple mastectomy and radiotherapy is a well established and generally safe form of treatment for breast cancer. It does, however, involve total breast loss and a high dose of radiation. There is a growing tendency to question the need for the use of both these treatments. Both have a role in the treatment of breast cancer but in the future their combined use may only be appropriate for a small subgroup of patients.

References

Aitken, D.R. & Minton, J.P. (1983) Complications associated with mastectomy. *Surg. Clins. North Am.*, *63*, 1331–1352.

Beatty, J.D., Robinson, G.V., Zaia, J.A. et al (1983) A prospective analysis of nosocomial wound infection after mastectomy. *Arch. Surg.*, *118*, 1421–1424.

Breast Cancer Symposium (1969) Points in the practical management of breast cancer. *Br. J. Surg.*, *56*, 782–796.

Brismar, B. & Ljungdahl, I. (1983) Postoperative lymphoedema after treatment of breast cancer. *Acta. Chir. Scand.*, *149*, 687–689.

Britton, R.C. & Nelson, P.A. (1962) Causes and treatment of post-mastectomy lymphoedema of the arm. *J. Am. Med. Ass.*, *180*, 95–102.

Cancer Research Campaign Working Party (1980) Cancer Research Campaign (King's/Cambridge) trial for early breast cancer. *Lancet, ii,* 55–60

Del Regato, J.A. (1971) Radiotherapy as a post-operative surgical adjuvant in the management of cancer of the breast. *Radiology*, *98*, 695–698.

Easson, E.C. (1969) Post-operative radiotherapy in breast cancer. In: *Prognostic factors in breast cancer.* ed. Forrest, A.P.M. & Kunkler, P.B. Edinburgh: Churchill Livingstone.

Ferguson, D.J., Sutton, H.G. & Dawson P.J. (1984) Late effects of adjuvant radiotherapy for breast cancer. *Cancer, 54,* 2319–2323.

Fisher, B., Redmond, C., Fisher, E.R. and participating NSABP investigators (1980) The contribution of recent NSABP clinical trials of primary breast cancer therapy to an understanding of tumour biology – an overview of findings. *Cancer, 46,* 1009–1025.

Halsted, W.S. (1894) The results of operations for the cure of cancer of the breast performed at the John Hopkins Hospital from June 1889 to January 1894. *Ann. Surg.*, *20*, 497–555.

Krohn, I.T., Cooper, D.R. & Bassett, J.G. (1982) Radical mastectomy: thick vs thin skin flaps. *Arch. Surg.*, *117*, 760–763.

Lacour, J., Monique, L.E., Caceres, E. et al. (1983) Radical mastectomy versus radical mastectomy plus internal mammary dissection: ten year results of an international cooperative trial in breast cancer. *Cancer, 51,* 1941–1943.

Langlands, A.O., Souter, W.A., Samuel, E. & Redpath, A.T. (1977) Radiation osteitis following irradiation for breast cancer. *Clin. Radiol., 28,* 93–96.

Lewis, D. & Reinhoff, W.F. (1932) A study of results of operations for the cure of cancer of the breast performed at the Johns Hopkins Hospital from 1889–1931. *Ann. Surg., 95,* 336–400.

Maguire, G.P., Lee, E.G., Bevington, D.J. et al (1978) Psychiatric problems in the first year after mastectomy. *Br. Med. J., 1,* 963–965.

McWhirter, R. (1948) The value of simple mastectomy and radiotherapy in the treatment of carcinoma of the breast. *Br. J. Radiol., 21,* 599–610.

Morris, T. (1979) Psychological adjustment to mastectomy. *Cancer Treat. Rev., 6,* 41–61.

Moxley, J.H. III, Allegra, J.C., Henney, J. & Muggia, F. (1980) Treatment of primary breast cancer. Summary of the National Institutes of Health Consensus Development Conference. *J. Am. Med. Ass., 244,* 797–800.

Roberts, M.M., Furnival, I.G. & Forrest, A.P.M. (1972) The morbidity of mastectomy. *Br. J. Surg., 59,* 301–302.

Say, C.C. & Donegan, W. (1974) A biostatistical evaluation of complications from mastectomy. *Surg. Gynecol. Obstet., 138,* 370–376.

Vana, J., Bedwani, R., Mettlin, C. & Murphy, G.P. (1981) Trends in diagnosis and management of breast cancer in the U.S.: From the surveys of the American College of Surgeons. *Cancer, 48,* 1043–1052.

11 Subcutaneous Mastectomy

Christopher Hinton & Iain Muir

To a woman with breast cancer the loss of a breast is second only in importance to the risk of her death. Surgeons have, therefore, long been turning their attention to looking for more conservative means of managing breast cancer so that the breast may be conserved or reconstructed. No study has ever shown that more conservative local measures result in an increased risk of death from breast cancer. In Nottingham in 1975 we began to offer young women the choice of having their breast cancer treated by the technique of subcutaneous mastectomy with subsequent subcutaneous prosthetic implant. The purpose of a subcutaneous mastectomy is to allow the woman the confidence of looking normal under her normal clothes without the necessity for her to wear any external prosthesis. We have been careful not to suggest to women undergoing subcutaneous mastectomy that they are likely to have a normal appearance to their unclothed breasts. This method of treatment is not suitable for every woman. There are limitations both from the nature of the tumour and the patient's breast. Tumours involving overlying skin requiring excision of large areas of skin are unsuitable for treatment in this fashion, as are women with very large or pendulous breasts, since no suitable prosthesis is available.

Technique

Through an incision in the submammary fold, the whole breast disc, including axillary tail, is excised as in simple mastectomy. The skin flaps are of the same thickness as in simple mastectomy, and may be produced by blunt dissection. Sharp dissection is, however, required to divide the major breast ducts beneath the nipple. Marking sutures should be placed at the nipple area and the axillary tail on the excised breast tissue to orientate the specimen for the pathologist. The wound is closed in layers over suction drainage and a compression dressing is applied. After removal of sutures, patients are asked to massage the retained breast skin with moisturizing cream to maintain maximum mobility. They are supplied with a temporary external prosthesis and once initial scarring and reaction has settled, usually at three to six months, they are offered breast reconstruction by the subcutaneous insertion of a silicone prosthesis.

Results of treatment by subcutaneous mastectomy
In order to assess the use of subcutaneous mastectomy for operable breast cancer, we have compared a series of 70 patients treated between 1975 and 1980 by subcutaneous mastectomy, with a group of 173 women in the same age range who had been treated by simple mastectomy over the same period of time. The minimum follow-up for these women was 30 months with a median of 56 months. Since this is not a controlled trial we have compared the groups when stratified according to prognostic factors determined at the time of mastectomy (Haybittle et al, 1982). We have been unable to show any difference in overall survival rate between those patients treated by subcutaneous or simple mastectomy (Fig. 11.1) (Hinton et al, 1984).

Figure 11.1 Survival of patients undergoing simple (SM) or subcutaneous (SCM) mastectomy: stratification by index of prognostic factors. There are no significant differences within each prognostic group.

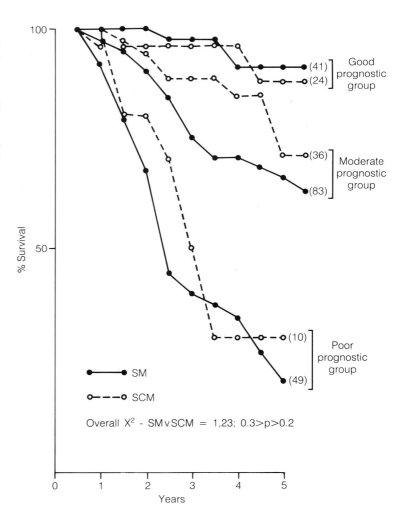

The complications of subcutaneous mastectomy

1 *Complications of the primary procedure*

The operative complications of subcutaneous mastectomy are those of any operation, the main problems being haemorrhage and haematoma formation. An attempt to avoid these is made by careful haemostasis and the use of adequate suction drainage.

In the immediate postoperative period, the main complication of the procedure has been flap ischaemia. In our series of 128 patients flap ischaemia has been seen in 24. In most of these this has amounted to small areas of superficial necrosis adjacent to the scar or in the nipple, though 2 have required conversion to simple mastectomy following necrosis of the large part of the flap and 2, although settling without further surgery, lost too much skin to permit implantation. Three factors are thought to contribute to the development of flap ischaemia:

   (i) The size of the breast itself may be a contributory factor as this is a direct determinant of the size of the skin flap.

   (ii) The thickness of the skin flap as fashioned at mastectomy.

   (iii) The presence of previous surgical scars.

The first of these has not been a major problem in our series as women with large, pendulous breasts have been excluded on the basis of there being little likelihood of a reasonable cosmetic result. When postmastectomy flap ischaemia was compared to the size of prosthesis later inserted there was no relationship between breast size and flap ischaemia.

Surgical technique is of great importance in determining the thickness of the skin flap, particularly in the nipple area where sharp dissection may take the plane of dissection very close to the skin. Apart from the four flap necroses, lesser degrees of superficial ischaemia have occurred particularly around the nipple area and, despite the dramatic appearance in these cases, recovery is the rule though subsequent reconstruction may be adversely affected.

The presence of previous surgical scars on the breast can be a problem, particularly if recent, and one of the patients who had to be converted to simple mastectomy had shortly before undergone excision biopsy of her carcinoma. Usually we avoid this by use of Trucut needle biopsy (Chapter 1); however, when an open biopsy had to be undertaken we have undertaken subcutaneous mastectomy through an extension of the previous biopsy wound. The ultimate appearances after subcutaneous implant in two patients on which this was performed were good.

2 *Local recurrence*

The only theoretical objection to subcutaneous mastectomy is

Figure 11.2
Local recurrences in patients who had simple (SM) or subcutaneous (SCM) mastectomy. Again there are no significant differences in the rate of local recurrence once stratification has been carried out according to prognostic factors.

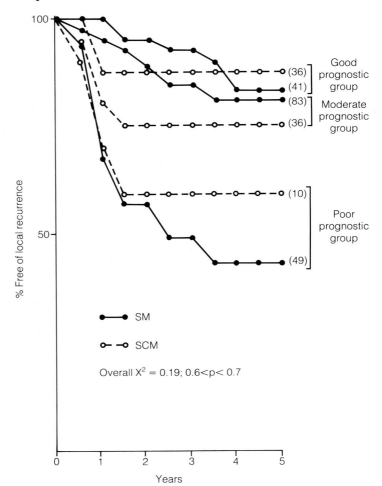

that the preservation of the skin of the breast and the nipple might lead to an incidence of incomplete excision and an increased incidence, therefore, of local recurrence. When the above patients, treated by subcutaneous mastectomy, were compared with the control group treated by simple mastectomy, we were able to show no significant difference in the incidence of local recurrence when patients were stratified according to prognostic factors (Fig. 11.2), and it therefore appears that when patients are carefully selected, and those with tumours known to be greater than 4 cm or with obvious skin involvement are excluded, the procedure can safely be performed without increasing the risk of local recurrence.

Two specific problems do occur in relation to subcutaneous mastectomy and local recurrence. Firstly, early local recurrence. In these patients early aggressive disease which recurs locally may require conversion to simple mastectomy and thus preclude the insertion of a subcutaneous prosthesis. Of the 128 patients treated by subcutaneous mastectomy in this unit, 4 have developed early recurrence such that reconstruction was inappropriate. In all of these patients completeness of excision was doubtful and it is now our custom in these cases where the pathologist is unsure of the completeness of excision (especially at the nipple) to administer postoperative prophylactic irradiation.

The second problem relating to local recurrence, is the possibility that the presence of the subcutaneous prosthesis may cause difficulty in the diagnosis of local recurrence. This may be because the recurrence is beneath the prosthesis and so remains occult, or because confusion arises in attributing fibrous or foreign body reactions to the prosthesis and local recurrence. Neither of these two factors have proved to be a problem in practice although foreign body reactions to the prosthesis have, on occasion, required excision to exclude the presence of local recurrence. It should be stressed that foreign body reactions to the intact prosthesis are extremely rare. However, if a prosthesis envelope is damaged and the gel leaks out foreign body reaction may be very marked.

Local recurrences in the region of the prosthesis are dealt with in the same fashion as they would be in patients with simple mastectomy, i.e. small localized recurrences are excised under local or general anaesthetic and multiple or widespread 'field change' local reaction is treated with radiotherapy. It should be noted that the presence of a prosthesis does not affect the administration of radiotherapy and the prosthesis itself is not affected by irradiation.

Technique of insertion of the silicone prosthesis

The procedure for the insertion of a prosthesis is simple. At approximately six months after subcutaneous mastectomy, the patient is readmitted to hospital and under general anaesthetic the old wound is opened and the subcutaneous plane developed. This is a loose fibrous layer between the skin flaps and pectoralis major. It has no significant blood vessels. The plane is extended and the flap stretched so that the prosthesis can be inserted beneath it. The prosthesis is inserted using a 'no touch technique' and the wound is closed in two layers.

The results of implanting subcutaneous silicone mammary prostheses have been good (Muir et al, 1985). Of 102 patients, 23 have had an excellent result, i.e. good shape and position nude (Fig. 11.3); 50 a good result, i.e. breasts indistinguishable when a bra is worn; 11 satisfactory, i.e. minimal padding required to produce normal appearance when patients fully clad; 7 patients had poor results with respect to size and position; 4 prostheses fell out due to wound breakdown.

Figure 11.3
Eight years post-
subcutaneous
mastectomy with
silicone implant: a
result classified as
excellent.

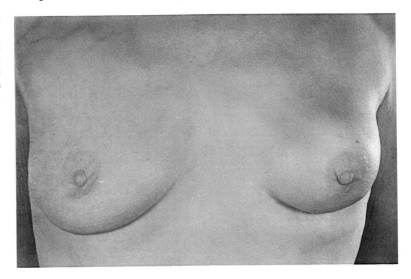

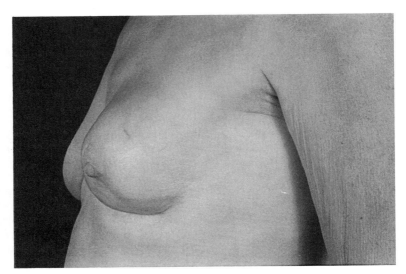

Complications of implantation

1 *Wound breakdown*

Wound breakdown is the major problem here and occurred in 5 of 102 prostheses inserted. All these losses occurred in patients who developed flap ischaemia after subcutaneous mastectomy; however, the fact that 3 out of 4 had a successful subsequent implant suggests that faulty technique may have been involved as well as ischaemia. We emphasize the need to dissect and stretch the skin flap to ensure that the wound can be closed without tension. It is also necessary to perform a two-layer closure of the wound, the first layer is in loose fibrous tissue which develops between skin and muscle after subcutaneous mastectomy. This is closed with interrupted chromic catgut, then subcuticular dexon is used in the skin. Haemorrhage and sepsis have not been troublesome. Antibiotics are not given routinely.

2 *Capsule formation*

Capsule contraction is the commonest complication of silicone implantation and in some degree it affects 75% of our patients. A capsule of fibrous tissue develops around all implanted silicone prostheses. In about 20%, this is thin and does not affect the shape or consistency of the prosthesis, but in the remainder thickening and contracture of the capsule takes place as is shown by hardening of the prosthesis and development of a more spherical shape. Two women in our series had such tight capsules that they developed pain in the region of the prosthesis.

At insertion of the prosthesis, several precautions are taken to minimize capsular contracture. We ensure that all powder is removed from the gloves of those participating in the procedure and that the prosthesis is handled as little as possible. After being removed from its sterile container, the prosthesis is rinsed in sterile saline solution and subsequently is only held in a sterile gauze swab before being carefully slid into the subcutaneous space prepared. The upper flap is elevated using Littlewood's forceps to prevent the prosthesis coming into contact with the patient's skin.

The management of capsular contracture depends on its severity. The great majority are amenable to 'closed rupture' (Fig. 11.4), i.e. the implanted breast is forcibly squeezed between the surgeon's hands until the rupture of the capsule can be heard or felt. The process can be repeated in more than one plane until satisfactory shape and consistency are obtained. Twenty-eight of our patients have required no closed rupture over a period of 106 patient years. The majority, however, appear to benefit from closed rupture at their yearly follow-up appointments. We have noticed that when a patient massages the implanted breast for a few minutes each day that capsule contraction is diminished.

Occasionally a capsule becomes so well developed that closed rupture is not possible or is too uncomfortable for the patient. Under these circumstances we offer patients 'open capsulotomy' under general anaesthetic. The patient is anaesthetized and a final attempt is made to perform a closed rupture. If this is unsuccessful the submammary wound is reopened taking care not to damage the prosthesis. The prosthesis is then delivered and the smooth fibrous capsule is divided in its equatorial plane using a No. 15 blade. The

Figure 11.4
Closed rupture being
undertaken in the
breast clinic.

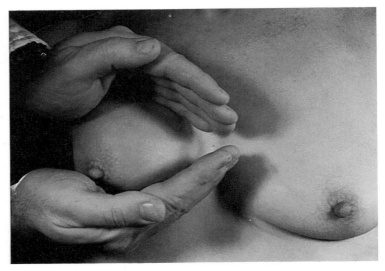

subcutaneous space is then stretched, the prosthesis reinserted with 'no touch' technique and the wound closed in two layers. In all, 16 patients have required open capsulotomy in a follow-up period of 40 patient years. Open capsulotomy does not protect against further capsular contracture and we have noticed that there is a higher incidence of wound sepsis after this procedure. Wound sepsis under these circumstances is always accompanied by loss of prosthesis, so we now reserve open capsulotomy only for the most severe cases of capsular contracture.

3 *Size and position*
Seven of our patients have poor results due to inappropriate size and position of the prosthesis. We have tried to gauge the size of implant by weighing the excised breast but this has not always given a good result. Initially, the tendency was for too small a prosthesis to be inserted, but increasing experience has diminished the problem. We suggest that a better estimate of implant size may be made by measuring the volume of the excised breast by water displacement or by using trial prostheses at the time of implantation.

Positioning of the prosthesis has not been a great problem and has improved with experience. However, it is worth mentioning that the lower skin flap should not be raised when inserting the prosthesis. If the subcutaneous mastectomy has been accomplished through an incision in the submammary fold, raising the lower flap at insertion of the prosthesis will certainly lead to the implant being too low. We have satisfactorily replaced prostheses for some women who have been dissatisfied with its size and position.

Prospects for further improvement

Ideally, a silicone implant should be placed at the same time as the patient undergoes subcutaneous mastectomy and this has been practised (Ward and Edwards, 1983). The procedure is complicated, however, by a high incidence of early loss of prosthesis, up to 20%, attributable to both flap ischaemia and haematoma formation. There is need, therefore, for a means of detecting flap ischaemia at the time of subcutaneous mastectomy in order to identify those patients who may or may not be safely implanted at the first operation. The use of xenon clearance measurements for the upper flap may be a suitable means.

Recent advances are reported from the USA using a polyurethane-covered silicone prosthesis (Herman, 1984). This device has a very fine meshwork of polyurethane fibres adherent to the envelope of the prosthesis and its insertion is accompanied by a very low rate of capsular contracture. Patient fibroblasts are said to invade the interstices of the polyurethane coating thus spreading the load of the device over a larger area of tissue when compared with the localized stresses engendered in the capsule around a smooth walled prosthesis. We have not yet been able to try out polyurethane-covered prostheses but the results from the USA are encouraging.

Conclusion

Subcutaneous mastectomy is a safe and effective way of treating primary breast cancer and permits the later insertion of a subcutaneous silicone prosthesis. The techniques are well within the capabilities of a general surgeon and do not demand a lot of operating time. The silicone implants lead to problems themselves but these are mostly minor and easily dealt with in the outpatient department. The development of the polyurethane prosthesis in the USA gives hope that capsular contraction around an implant may be avoided once this device is more readily available.

References

Haybittle, J.L., Blamey, R.W., Elston, C.W. et al (1982) A prognostic index in primary breast cancer. *Br. J. Cancer*, *42*, 361–366.

Herman, S. (1984) The Meme implant. *Plast. Reconstr. Surg.*, *73*, 411–414.

Hinton, C.P., Doyle, P.J., Blamey, R.W. et al (1984) Subcutaneous mastectomy for primary operable breast cancer. *Br. J. Surg.*, *71*, 469–472.

Muir, I.M., Hinton, C.P., Williams, M.R. & Blamey, R.W. (1986) Subcutaneous mastectomy with delayed insertion of subcutaneous silicone mammary prosthesis. The results of 8 years' experience. In press.

Ward, D.C. & Edwards, M.J. (1983) Early results of subcutaneous mastectomy with immediate silicone prosthetic implant for carcinoma of the breast. *Br. J. Surg.*, *70*, 651–653.

12 Excision with Irradiation

David Morgan

The past few decades have seen a number of large clinical trials comparing one form of locoregional treatment for breast cancer with another, but the greatest value of these trials has been not what they have demonstrated about the initial local therapy of breast cancer, but what they have taught us about the systemic nature of the disease. It appears that the great majority of patients who present with apparently local or locoregional disease already have established, if clinically undetectable, metastatic spread and so no matter how radical the local treatment that is given, these patients eventually succumb to the disease. The doubt cast in recent years on the value of extended local treatments when compared to simple mastectomy alone as primary therapy, has led in turn to the questioning of whether complete removal of the breast is itself not unnecessarily mutilating. Increasing interest has developed, at first in medical circles, but now in the popular media, in breast-conserving treatments (Fig. 12.1).

These, of course, are not new, having been applied as early as 1924 by Keynes who performed local excision of tumour followed by radium needle implant. His work, because it employed solid radioactive isotopes, was interrupted by war and never resumed. The next developments in this field occurred in France when Baclesse, even in the days of orthovoltage equipment, was treating breast cancer by protracted courses of irradiation to the whole breast and lymph node regions. His work was continued, using supervoltage equipment (cobalt-60) by Calle and other French groups, and interest in this form of treatment has gradually spread round the world. Its impact on the English-speaking countries has probably been first really felt during the 1970s, and our group decided in 1979 to offer such treatment to younger patients, as an alternative to mastectomy. The choice of treatment has been the patient's, after being given the opportunity to discuss the options in detail, with both surgeon and radiotherapist. At the time of writing, over 150 patients have chosen to be treated by local excision of tumour followed by irradiation, and the first five years' experience has encouraged us to continue this policy. In this chapter the problems and complications that arise when patients are treated conservatively are discussed. Many of these are dissimilar to those that

Figure 12.1
Excellent result.
Treated by mega-
voltage boost.

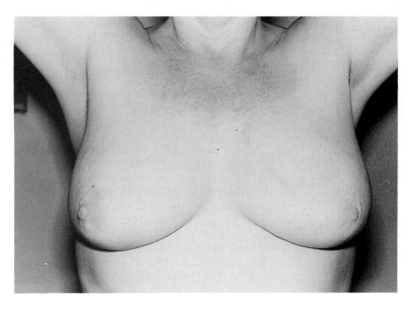

Figure 12.1 Excellent result. Treated by mega-voltage boost.

beset patients treated by mastectomy, but there is a lot of common ground. The main problem for all patients treated for breast cancer, by whatever method, is the probability of disease recurrence; the threat of this hangs over the patient for the rest of her life.

An immediate distinction is drawn here between locoregional and distant recurrence. As far as the latter is concerned, the problem is the same for patients treated by lumpectomy and irradiation as for those treated by mastectomy. These problems are discussed elsewhere.

Short-term problems

The immediate difficulties for the patients are those associated with any minor surgical procedure and with a course of radio-therapy. In our group, it is the policy to perform a staging double-node biopsy either at the time of lumpectomy, if the lesion has been confirmed as malignant by out-patient Trucut biopsy, or shortly afterwards. The low axillary and internal mammary nodes are sampled: this necessitates one or two extra incisions besides that performed for the lumpectomy. The scars should be healed before the radiotherapy begins, although, in fact, skin healing does not seem to be impaired by the irradiation. A 'lumpiness' often persists in the breast at the side of lumpectomy throughout the course of irradiation, caused by a degree of oedema and/or haematoma at the site of excision. This often feels hard and irregular like a cancer, but can be distinguished from residual malignancy by its gradual resolution, although this often does not occur until radiotherapy has been completed.

The problems associated with the radiotherapy are those of any course of irradiation. The inconvenience of attending the radiotherapy department daily for about six weeks is not least among these. In Nottingham, where most of our patients come from within a fairly small geographic area, this problem is less pronounced than it is in other parts of the country or the world.

The usual technique of irradiation in our department, as in many others, is to deliver 45 Gy over four and a half weeks to the whole breast by tangential opposed fields, followed by a 'boost' to the tumour bed. The full dose is delivered to the deep tissues, and the skin-sparing effort of megavoltage irradiation is employed to full advantage as no bolus is usually used. The lumpectomy site then receives a 'boost' of 15 Gy over a week and a half, often using a similar technique, but occasionally by other methods, such as by a 14 MeV electron beam. The actual treatment time each day is relatively short and does not usually cause great social inconvenience. Indeed, many patients are able to carry on working during their course of radiotherapy.

The majority of patients treated do not experience severe side-effects from their irradiation. A degree of skin reaction is universal, but this rarely amounts to more than a moderate erythema, followed by dry desquamation. Moist desquamation is unusual unless electrons, orthovoltage equipment or an iridium implant are used to deliver the boost—except in the infra-mammary sulcus in the pendulous breast, which often shows a small degree of this towards the end of the first phase of treatment; resolution occurs within two weeks or so.

Systemic side-effects from irradiation are also not a major problem: many patients experience a mild degree of malaise or fatigue, with a very few complaining of some nausea. In our department we have never known a patient need to interrupt treatment because of its side-effects, and, as mentioned above, many patients are able to continue with their work.

In many patients the irradiated skin shows a degree of dusky pigmentation that may persist for some months after the desquamation has finished, but this almost always eventually vanishes.

As the course of radiotherapy progresses, some patients experience a soreness in the breast that may resemble premenstrual discomfort. This can be a source of some concern, particularly as it sometimes persists for some months, and occasionally as long as a year. The cause of this discomfort is not clear, and it seems to be in no degree related to the severity of the acute skin reaction.

Very rarely the skin of the breast develops a degree of lymphoedema following radiotherapy giving a peau d'orange appearance, that may resemble diffuse local recurrence of malignancy (Fig. 12.2). The lymphoedema subsides over a period of a few months. Although, clinically, this problem is rarely detectable, some skin oedema is a very common feature mammographically, again usually resolving within a few months.

Figure 12.2
Slight peau d'orange
following breast irra-
diation. No evidence
of recurrence within
the breast.

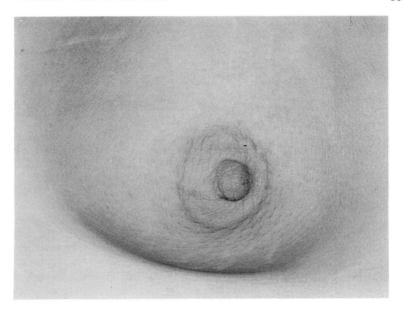

Problems in follow-up: the treated area

It is our policy to review patients one month after completing irradiation, then at three-monthly intervals for eighteen months, and six-monthly intervals thereafter. Useful though mammography is, clinical examination remains paramount.

Often, but not always, the irradiated breast undergoes a change of texture which is noticeable on palpation, becoming diffusely rather firmer throughout. The site of the tumour, to which an extra dose of irradiation has been delivered, may, in particular, become quite indurated. This induration may be difficult to distinguish from tumour recurrence, particularly for those inexperienced in examining such patients. Mammography is sometimes helpful in distinguishing such postirradiation change from tumour recurrence, but it is our policy to perform a Trucut needle biopsy whenever there is the slightest clinical doubt, as it is important that local recurrence be dealt with early.

Mammography is performed on a routine basis, firstly at six months after finishing treatment (to allow postirradiation changes to resolve), again six months later, and then yearly. The mammographic appearances of the irradiated breast require expert interpretation, but do sometimes give the first hint of local recurrence. When the mammographic evidence of recurrence is strong, even in the absence of clinical signs, a 'marker' biopsy is taken. On the other hand, a negative mammogram does not necessarily exclude disease recurrence and when there is clinical doubt early recourse to biopsy should be taken.

If local recurrence does occur, treatment is surgical. This will usually entail mastectomy; the occasional recurrence may be quite superficial and amenable to local excision, in the same way as 'spot recurrence' can be excised following mastectomy, with good long-term control in some cases (Chapter 16). The surgeons in our team have not found operating in an irradiated breast particularly difficult, and the wounds usually heal well.

The problems of lymph node and distant metastasis are essentially the same for these patients as for patients treated by mastectomy. It is our policy not to irradiate the regional nodes prophylactically following surgery, whether lumpectomy or mastectomy, whatever the histological status of the nodes may be. Node recurrence after lumpectomy is dealt with by surgery, irradiation, or systemic therapy in just the same way as after mastectomy.

The avoidance of axillary dissection and routine nodal irradiation is an important factor in reducing morbidity, especially lymphoedema of the arm and breast. This topic has recently been the subject of a detailed review (Yarnold, 1984).

Radiation damage to normal tissues can occasionally cause problems during the first year after treatment. The discomfort often experienced in the breast and/or chest wall has been alluded to, and is usually self-limiting. Very rarely, minor trauma can result in the fracture of an irradiated rib. This is painful and rather more slow to heal than a fracture of a normal rib. No specific treatment is indicated other than simple analgesia.

The tangential radiation fields that cover the whole breast inevitably encompass a certain volume of lung tissue. If, as in our unit, no specific attempt is made to include the regional node areas in the treatment volume (particularly the internal mammary nodes), the amount of lung irradiated will not be great, and postirradiation pulmonary problems should not be common. In fact, we have never yet seen a case of symptomatic radiation pneumonitis. For this reason, and because their value in screening for asymptomatic metastatic disease is so little, we do not perform routine chest X-rays as part of our follow-up, and so cannot comment on the incidence of asymptomatic radiological pulmonary changes.

The effects of radiation on other normal tissues are of prime interest when lumpectomy and radiotherapy are being considered. If this form of treatment is to be acceptable as an alternative to mastectomy, it must, first and foremost, give good cosmetic results, as it is the hope of a cosmetically less devastating result that is the only advantage of this form of therapy.

Most authors report that, in fact, the cosmetic results of whole breast irradiation are nowadays very good. When employing this treatment it is not usually desirable to achieve the full 'radical' dose at the skin surface, as mentioned earlier; as well as sparing the patient the unpleasantness of a severe early skin reaction, this results in a diminution in the incidence and severity of late skin changes. Such skin stigmata can occur, usually only in the

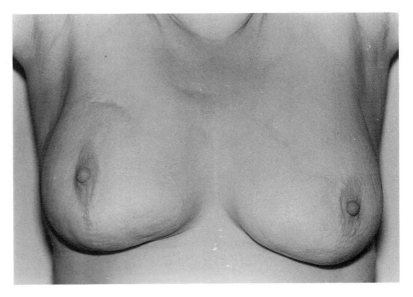

area that receives a booster dose, and to some extent they can be minimized by careful planning of the radiotherapy technique and fractionation. Thus, when this form of treatment was first used regularly in our department, it was usual to deliver the boost by orthovoltage equipment concurrently with the last week or two of the whole-breast irradiation on the linear accelerator. This technique produced a number of rather ugly areas of skin (Fig. 12.3) at the booster site, as might be expected from modern radiobiological evidence. To deliver the booster consecutively (as we now do) seems a better policy, and one that gives far better results as far as the skin is concerned.

The same considerations apply to the breast tissue itself, with concurrent boosts giving less satisfactory results than consecutive treatment. In particular, the patients given a concurrent boost often develop a hard fibrous mass in the breast at the site of the original tumour, and this causes problems in clinical interpretation. As mentioned earlier, we advocate a policy of early, and if necessary, repeated biopsy of such areas. Naturally, these fibrotic areas also represent a less satisfactory result from the point of view of resemblance to the normal breast.

There are, besides the radiation effects, two other causes of cosmetic imperfection associated with this unit's technique of treatment that may not be seen elsewhere, where other methods are used.

Firstly, as mentioned previously, it is our policy to perform node biopsies as a staging procedure, as part of a long-term study of prognostic factors in breast cancer. This necessitates one or two extra incisions, besides that through which the lumpectomy is performed, depending on the site of the tumour. An internal mammary node and a low axillary node are removed for histo-pathological examination. If an additional axillary incision is performed, the resulting scar rarely worries the patient in later years, as it is not readily visible. On the other hand, the scar resulting from the internal mammary biopsy is often a cause of some concern, as it is an area that many ladies often leave uncovered, and scars in this area unfortunately often look quite ugly. (By comparison, the scar of the lumpectomy is often quite unnoticeable after a few months.) On a small number of occasions these internal mammary biopsy scars have required re-excision at a later date.

Secondly, the technique of irradiation that we employ requires marking on the patients' skin of two points to enable the linear accelerator head and couch to be set in position each day, one being used for the front pointer of the set and one for the back pointer. Because of the duration of the treatment it is our practice to tattoo these points with a small dot of india ink. In effect, this produces one spot at the medial edge of the breast and one at the lateral. When the boost is also given by linear accelerator (as is our usual practice), two further spots are also tattooed. The majority of patients find these tattoos no cause for concern, but a few are very unhappy with them, in which case they can be simply removed under local anaesthetic using a dermatological punch biopsy. This, of course, also leaves a small scar, but one of a more 'natural' colour, which is usually acceptable to the patient.

There is one other observation relating to the irradiated breast that we have encountered that is worthy of mention. Two ladies treated by lumpectomy and radiotherapy have, at a later date, decided to conceive. This has been after a long discussion with the medical staff, and both ladies have been fully aware of the degree of uncertainty relating to their long-term prognosis. Both these patients were, in fact, under the age of 30 at the time of diagnosis of breast cancer. Both went through normal preg-nancies and deliveries, and both decided to breast-feed. The untreated breast underwent the usual degree of hypertrophy during pregnancy and lactation, whereas the irradiated breast did not enlarge, nor lactate, yet in one case developed stretch marks. The unirradiated breast was able to produce an adequate supply of milk in both cases.

Other problems
While concentrating on the treated breast, it must not be forgotten that the contralateral breast is at risk of developing a new primary tumour. It is generally held that, in patients treated for cancer of one breast, this risk is greater than the risk of a tumour arising in a breast of a lady who has not had cancer, but an exact figure for such a risk is not easy to determine. It has certainly been our experience that contralateral tumours occur

relatively frequently, and possibly more frequently in the patients we have treated by lumpectomy and radiotherapy than in patients treated by mastectomy. However, a number of factors are involved that make comparison difficult.

Firstly, the patients treated by lumpectomy have tended to be the younger ones. It has been previously reported that younger patients are more likely to develop bilateral tumours. Also, the policy of performing regular mammography, when the untreated breast is always examined as well as the treated one, may increase the detection rate, and it has certainly been the case that some of the contralateral tumours we have seen have been detected mammographically before becoming clinically manifest.

The other possibility is that the contralateral tumours are radiation-induced. This seems unlikely, but not altogether impossible. We have estimated that the dose of irradiation to the contralateral breast during a course of radiotherapy to one breast by our technique is, very roughly, 3 Gy for the medial breast tissues, and 0.25 Gy for the lateral tissues. Yet, of the few contralateral tumours we have seen, as many have occurred in outer quadrants as in inner quadrants. It is also widely accepted that radiation-induced carcinomas (as opposed to haematological malignancies) have a latent period of over ten years, in which case the contralateral tumours we have seen should not be radiogenic.

The above assumptions may be wrong: only detailed further follow-up can furnish data on whether the contralateral tumour incidence is related to the treatment or to the nature of the disease. Even so, it must be remembered that the risk of a contralateral tumour remains almost negligible by comparison with that of developing secondary disease from the original tumour. Lastly, just as an increased risk of radiation-induced contralateral breast tumours cannot be excluded, the possibility remains that radiotherapy induces tumours at sites other than the breast (as a result of radiation scattering). Our patients have not been followed up long enough to make any assessment of this, nor is there any published data that even attempts to quantify this risk. It is clear that, if at all real, this risk is very small, and almost insignificant when compared to the hazards of having suffered from primary breast cancer itself.

Conclusion

Treatment of breast cancer by 'excision/irradiation' is being employed increasingly—not least because of the demand for such treatment by patients themselves. While precise data on how it compares with mastectomy in terms of survival are not available, evidence is accumulating to suggest that any difference that there may be in this respect is unlikely to be very large. Its cosmetic result is far preferable to most patients, the local recurrence rate is low, and undesirable side-effects and complications can be kept at an acceptably low level; but patients treated in this way must be followed-up meticulously.

<table>
<tr><td>Controversies
and Future
Developments</td><td>

• Radiotherapeutic dose and number of fractions.
• Whether to carry out simultaneous prophylactic node irradiation.
• The identification of cases unsuitable for this form of treatment.
• The use of mammography and fine-needle aspiration in follow-up.
• Whether wide excision of the primary tumour is necessary.</td></tr>
</table>

Further reading

Calle, R., Pilleron, J.P., Schlienger, P. & Vilcoq, J.R. (1978) Conservative management of operable breast cancer: Ten years experience at the Fondation Curie. *Cancer*, *42*, 2045–2053.

Harris, J.R. & Hellman, S. (1983) Primary radiation therapy for early breast cancer. *Cancer*, *52*, 2547–2552.

Yarnold, J.R. (1984) Selective avoidance of lymphatic irradiation in the conservative management of breast cancer. *Radiotherapy and Oncology*, *2*, 79–91.

13 Adjuvant Systemic Therapy

Roger Blamey

The side-effects of adjuvant therapies are, of course, the same as those of the therapies used for advanced disease. Cytotoxic chemotherapy has unpleasant side-effects (Chapter 22). Unless its use carries a clear advantage in terms of survival it should not be used for adjuvant therapy. Endocrine therapy in the form of tamoxifen, on the other hand, has negligible side-effects; the use of this adjuvant therapy may be advised.

Cytotoxic chemotherapy
With cytotoxic chemotherapy the side-effects are certainly unpleasant. A study at the Royal Marsden Hospital demonstrated that 62% of patients receiving combination chemotherapy as adjuvant treatment described it as 'very unpleasant' and one patient in three voluntarily added that 'it could never be gone through again'. The Royal Marsden workers concluded that 'such treatment is only justified if there is a substantial survival advantage'. A recent paper adds to the usual list of side-effects a list of viral infections contracted by women on adjuvant chemotherapy.

Whether there is any survival advantage is debatable. The great majority of randomized trials of cytotoxic therapy compared with an untreated control group (and certainly those carried out in the UK) show no significant survival advantage, although the well quoted study of Bonadonna (1985) does show a 10–12% advantage at five years. Several studies, however, show a trend towards a better survival in the adjuvant-treated group. Peto (1985) has reported that the combination of all known trials shows a small survival advantage, more pronounced in the subgroup with 1–3 nodes positive at mastectomy in premenopausal women. Why this latter group should show this is not clear, since survival without adjuvant chemotherapy, tumour histological grade etc. are closely similar to those in women of other age groups with breast cancer.

What is clear is that there is no 'substantial' survival advantage. The trials have also failed to answer the more important question of whether adjuvant treatment confers advantage over a group which the clinician ensures receives the same cytotoxic therapy during the course of their secondary disease. If no such advantage is demonstrable then all clinicians will surely hold back such treatment until it is required.

The best way to avoid the side-effects of adjuvant cytotoxic therapy is not to use it. In the absence of a demonstrated substantial survival advantage of adjuvant chemotherapy over chemotherapy reserved and applied if thought necessary in the secondary phase, I believe that the present application of adjuvant chemotherapy is unjustified.

Endocrine therapy

The case for adjuvant endocrine therapy is different. Trials of various endocrine therapies have sometimes shown a survival advantage (Baum et al, 1985), and sometimes not (Cole, 1970). What is absolutely clear, and predictable, is that there is a mean lengthening of the disease-free interval. To keep a woman free of symptoms and worry for a longer period before secondary symptoms emerge is itself an advantage. Tamoxifen with its lack of side-effects may be given to patients likely to develop secondary disease—possibly those node-positive or, better, identified by a prognostic index (Haybittle et al, 1982). Logically this treatment should be only applied to ER-positive tumours. This has been demonstrated by the results of the Danish cooperative group; in their trial only patients with ER-positive tumours derived the benefit of the lengthening of the symptom-free interval.

Controversies and Future Developments

- The whole subject remains controversial and exact analysis is required of the total months of benefit per 1000 women and the misery produced among them by the side-effects.
- The place of ER assays in advising adjuvant endocrine therapy.

Further reading

Baum, M. et al (1985) Controlled trial of tamoxifen as single adjuvant agent in management of early breast cancer: analysis at six years by Nolvadex Adjuvant Trial Organisation. *Lancet, i,* 836–839.

Bonadonna, G. (1985) Adjuvant CMF chemotherapy in operable breast cancer: ten years later. *Lancet* (letter), 27th April 1985, p. 976.

Cole, M.P. (1970) Prophylactic compared with therapeutic X-ray artificial menopause. In: *Clinical Management of Advanced Breast Cancer*, Proceedings of Second Tenovus Workshop, ed. Joslin, C.A.F. & Gleave, E.N. Cardiff: Alpha-Omega, pp. 2–11.

Haybittle, J.L., Blamey, R.W., Elston, C.W. et al (1982) A prognostic index in primary breast cancer. *Br. J. Cancer, 45,* 361.

Palmer, B.V., Walsh, G.A., McKinna, J.A. & Greening, W.P. (1980) Adjuvant chemotherapy for breast cancer: side effects and quality of life. *Br. Med. J., 2,* 1594.

Peto, R. (1985) Cytotoxic chemotherapy in breast cancer. *Lancet* (letter), 19th January 1985, p. 162.

Rose, C., Thorpe, S.M., Anderson, K.W. et al (1985) Beneficial effect of adjuvant tamoxifen therapy in primary breast cancer patients with high oestrogen receptor values. *Lancet, i,* 16–19.

14 Locally Advanced Breast Cancer

Michael Williams

Fifteen per cent of patients presenting to our unit with carcinoma of the breast had clinical features which classified their primary tumours as locally advanced. It was Haagenson and Stout in 1943 who first established operability guidelines for patients presenting in this way. These guidelines were based on their observations that certain grave features predicted poor results when patients were subjected to radical surgery. They later confirmed their findings when reporting a series of patients deemed inoperable on these criteria. The local recurrence rate after radical surgery in this series was 49% and only one patient could be considered a 5 year 'cure'. Thus, despite the technical feasibility of radical surgery in many cases with locally advanced breast cancer, the development of local recurrence or metastases is unacceptably high for this form of therapy to be used. Since Haagenson and Stout reported their findings, many different treatment regimens have been evaluated as first-line therapies for locally advanced tumours. Until recently, radical radiotherapy has been the most frequently employed of these regimes. A local response rate of approximately 60% can be expected. However, the majority of these patients develop both locally progressive and metastatic disease within 18 months (Rubens et al, 1977; Langlands et al, 1980). Improved local control has been claimed with the use of supervoltage techniques at dose levels between 5000 and 8000 rads, but there is additional treatment morbidity including pulmonary fibrosis, skin necrosis and lymphoedema (Brufman et al, 1981).

To date no worthwhile survival advantage has been shown by combining more aggressive regimens, incorporating cytotoxic agents, with local radiotherapy as first-line therapy. Treatment morbidity is significantly increased when using these agents.

Clinical features and investigations

Locally advanced breast cancer may present in many different clinical guises (Figs 14.1 & 14.2). The features contributing toward the inoperability of these tumours are a combination of both size and fixation of the primary lesion and the extent of involvement of draining lymph nodes.

Tumours greater than 5 cm in diameter even when fully mobile have a high chance of local recurrence after radical surgery

Figure 14.1
Locally advanced
tumour showing peau
d'orange.

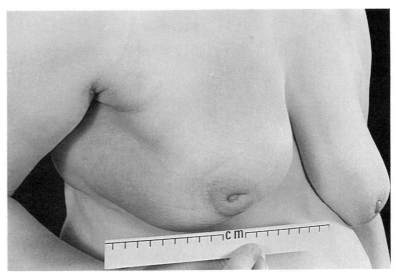

alone, with poor long-term survival. Smaller tumours when fixed to pectoral muscles are again untreatable by surgery alone. More dramatic features of advanced tumours include fungation or ulceration of skin and the presence of surrounding peau d'orange. Matting and fixation of axillary lymph nodes or involvement of supraclavicular nodes again render the primary tumour inoperable. Tumours presenting with these features are usually classified by their TNM stage—III, or stage IV when metastases are already clinically detectable.

Although diagnosis of locally advanced carcinoma is usually blatantly obvious on observation alone, histological confirmation is required in all cases prior to treatment. This can be achieved easily in the majority of cases by Trucut needle biopsy under local anaesthetic in the out-patient clinic.

The patient is fully examined to determine the extent of local disease and to identify any overt metastases. This initial assessment should also include careful measurement and documentation of all local disease so that a later response to treatment can be assessed accurately. Photography is often helpful in this respect. Haematological investigations include FBC, ESR and liver function tests; a chest X-ray and bone scan are performed to identify associated bone or pulmonary metastases. Hepatic and brain scans are requested only if clinically indicated.

With the development of oestrogen receptor assays, a method has become available by which some prediction of a later response to endocrine treatment can be made. These assays require attention to detail in rapid freezing of tumour tissue with liquid nitrogen immediately after the biopsy is performed. It is also necessary to carry out the biopsy under general anaesthetic,

Figure 14.2
Locally advanced
tumour with
ulceration.

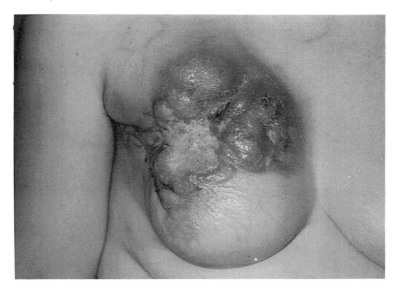

as an 'open' procedure, to provide sufficient tumour for analysis. Despite these technical difficulties, oestrogen receptors may adopt an increasingly important role in the management of advanced breast cancer in future years.

The clinical assessment of response

The UICC and British Breast Group (BBG) have laid down criteria by which an objective assessment of response to treatment can be made in advanced breast cancer. These criteria have provided a standard for the definition of a response so that it is now possible to compare different treatment regimens assessed on similar criteria both within and between series. The UICC require a 50% reduction in the size (bidimentional product) of measurable disease (e.g. locoregional disease) or objective signs of improvement at evaluable sites (e.g. bone or pulmonary metastases). The British Breast Group (1974) has recommended a minimum duration of remission of at least six months before disease is classified as responding. The time from starting treatment to tumour regression varies considerably between patients but a high proportion of patients destined to respond to endocrine manipulation will show evidence of tumour regression by three months. In some cases, however, disease may remain static for many months before a true response is seen. Mammographic assessment of primary tumour size prior to and throughout treatment may also help in the later evaluation of a response to therapy (Sauven et al, 1983).

The treatment of advanced breast cancer

Once the initial assessment has been completed, patients can be

Figure 14.3
Duration of remission
in responders to
Nolvadex therapy.

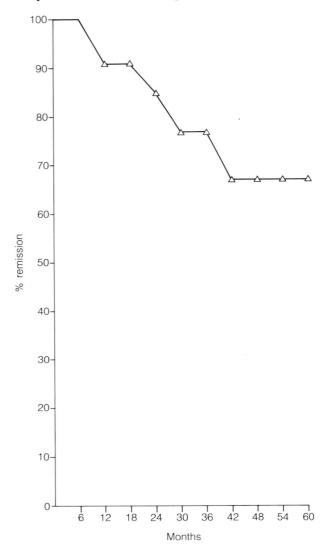

separated into those with no overt metastases and those in whom distant metastases are already clinically detectable. Clearly, in the latter group local treatments alone are not applicable. Systemic endocrine therapy is indicated to palliate both local disease and distant metastases simultaneously.

In the majority of patients with locally advanced carcinoma, the emergence of symptomatic metastases within a short time is inevitable and this forms the rationale behind the use of endocrine therapy as first-line treatment in this situation. In addition, holding the primary tumour in check using endocrine therapy is doing so without treatment morbidity.

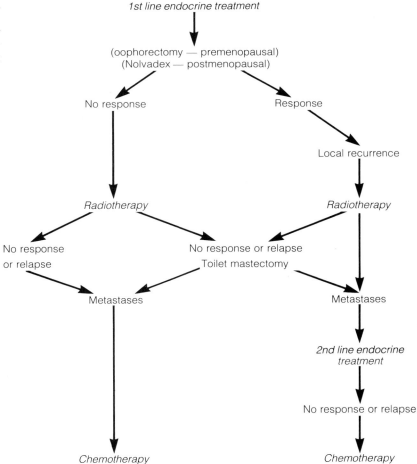

Figure 14.4
Suggested protocol
for treatment for
patients with locally
advanced breast
cancer.

1st line endocrine treatment

(oophorectomy — premenopausal)
(Nolvadex — postmenopausal)

No response   Response

Local recurrence

Radiotherapy   Radiotherapy

No response   No response or relapse
or relapse   Toilet mastectomy

Metastases   Metastases

2nd line endocrine
treatment

No response or relapse

Chemotherapy   Chemotherapy

If the disease progresses despite endocrine treatment, radiotherapy is employed locally as a secondary procedure. There is no
evidence that any delay so incurred reduces the response rate to
radiotherapy. Such a delay in employing radiotherapy will, in
any case, be short (2–3 months) in the face of progressing local
disease. When adopting this regimen of treatment, some patients
will be spared the side-effects of radiotherapy since they succumb
to disseminated disease or incidental illness (the majority of
patients are elderly) while the local tumour remains in response.

In our preliminary series of 51 postmenopausal women with
inoperable cancer of the breast initially with tamoxifen (Nolvadex 20 mg b.d.s.) alone, an objective response (UICC) was
observed in 40% of patients (Campbell et al, 1984). Seventy-five
per cent of responders remained in remission at a median follow
up of 36 months (Fig. 14.3). Patients, in whom tumour progressed

at two months or remained static at six months, received radiotherapy as a secondary procedure with a response rate of 66%. The median duration of this secondary response was 10 months.

In those patients relapsing after a response to endocrine therapy where disease is progressing despite radiotherapy, a second-line endocrine agent may occasionally be effective (e.g. megestrol acetate 160 mg b.d.s.). Finally, cytotoxic chemotherapy may have to be used. We do not routinely use cytotoxic therapy in the over-seventies because of the toxicity (Chapter 22) and symptomatic palliation is an alternative in this group.

Although, in general, patients presenting with locally advanced disease have a very poor prognosis, certain tumours may be associated with a relatively prolonged survival when compared with other rapidly growing, early metastasizing tumours. Typically, these patients present with long histories and are more often elderly, having withheld from seeking medical advice. In such patients 'toilet mastectomy' may control local fungation and ulceration if less aggressive alternative treatments have not been effective and prolonged survival is expected on clinical grounds.

A suggested protocol for treatment for patients with locally advanced breast cancer is shown in Fig. 14.4.

Conclusions
The only consistent finding from many series of patients presenting with locally advanced breast cancer is the consistently poor survival when patients are subjected to current treatments. However, therapy may improve the quality of life for patients presenting in this way. The realization that radical surgery cannot 'cure' locally advanced breast cancer has in itself reduced unnecessary morbidity associated with these procedures. The introduction of simple non-toxic forms of endocrine therapy, with radiotherapy reserved as a second-line treatment, provides effective palliation with few adverse side-effects for a high percentage of patients responding.

The assessment of response to treatment in local disease is a simple matter of measuring the primary tumour and this can be taken as a reflection of the total disease in that patient. In some cases, several months have to pass before any reliable decision to change therapy can be made. More accurate methods of assessing

Table 14.1

	ER-positive	ER-negative	No ER measurement
Response	12	7	4
No response	7	14	7

$0.2 > P > 0.1$

the total disease are required so that the treatments can be tailored to the individual patient. Despite the results from our series (Table 14.1), ER assays may provide some discrimination between those likely to respond or progress on endocrine therapy but are of no use when other treatments are employed. Possibly, in future years, only those patients with ER-positive primary tumours will be treated initially with endocrine therapy, patients with ER-negative tumour receiving radiotherapy as their first-line treatment.

Controversies and Future Developments

• The optimal methods of treatment will finally be worked out through clinical trials; ideally, however, locally advanced disease would be prevented by earlier detection.

References

British Breast Group (1974) Assessment of response to treatment in advanced breast cancer. *Lancet, ii*, 38–39.

Brufman, G., Weshler, Z., Prosnitz, L.R. & Fuks, Z. (1981) Treatment of locally advanced breast carcinoma with high dose external beam supervoltage radiotherapy. *Isr. J. Med. Sci., 17*, 940–945.

Campbell, F.C., Morgan, D.A.L., Bishop, H.M. et al (1984) The management of locally advanced carcinoma of the breast by Nolvadex (tamoxifen): A pilot study. *Clin. Oncol., 10*, 111–115.

Haagenson, C.D. & Stout, A.P. (1943) Carcinoma of the breast: criteria of operability. *Ann. Surg., 118*, 859–870.

Hayward, J.L., Carbonne, P.P., Hewson, J.C. et al (1977) Assessment of response to therapy in advanced breast cancer. *Cancer, 39*, 1289–1293.

Langlands, A.O., Forbes, J.F. & Tattersall, M.H.T. (1980) The treatment of locally advanced breast cancer. A discussion document. *Aust. Radiol., 24*, 307–310.

Rubens, R.D., Armitage, P., Winter, P.J., Toney, D. & Hayward, J.L. (1977) Prognosis in inoperable stage 3 carcinoma of the breast. *Europ. J. Cancer, 13*, 805–811.

Sauven, P., Grant, R. & Burn, I. (1983) The role of mammography in the evaluation of advanced breast cancer treated by initial endocrine therapy. *Br. J. Surg., 70*, 453–456.

15 Psychological Complications of Mastectomy

Peter Maguire

A substantial proportion of women who undergo mastectomy for breast cancer develop psychiatric morbidity. The nature of this morbidity, its recognition and treatment will be discussed.

Depressive illness

At least one in four women who undergo mastectomy develop a depressive illness (Morris, 1979; Maguire, 1984a). The woman reports that she has been feeling persistently low and miserable to an extent which represents a distinct departure from her normal mood. She finds she cannot distract herself out of it or be brought out of it by others. As well as this persistent low mood there are other symptoms of depression which may include: irritability, impaired concentration and forgetfulness, loss or increase in appetite, loss or increase in weight, loss of libido, loss of energy, repeated waking or early morning waking, agitation or retardation, feelings of hopelessness about the future, guilt, worthlessness, feeling a burden and suicidal ideas. This depressive illness usually has a marked effect on the patient's ability to function. The woman will report that she is finding it an increasing effort to cope with her chores or work. Indeed, she may fail to return to work despite being physically well. There may also be marked social withdrawal—the woman has stopped going out because she wants to avoid meeting other people and wishes to hide away from the world.

Anxiety states

A fifth of women are also at risk of developing an anxiety state (Maguire et al, 1978). They find themselves plagued by worry and cannot push these worries out of their minds or be distracted by others. They are unable to relax and feel constantly on edge and tense. They usually have considerable difficulty getting off to sleep because of these worries, feel increasingly irritable and notice that they find it hard to concentrate and make decisions. Commonly, physical symptoms like palpitations, sweating, headache and breathlessness, shakiness and tremor may be prominent. If they also suffer from over-breathing they may report numbness and parathesiae. It should be clear from the history that these symptoms of anxiety represent a distinct difference from the patient's normal behaviour even if they claim that they have always been 'worriers'.

The anxiety usually presents in this generalized way but sometimes agoraphobia develops. Anxiety is then triggered by fear of specific situations. For example, the patient becomes afraid of going out of the house alone. She fears that if she does she could collapse and even die. Such patients are often also fearful of going into shops, particularly supermarkets, in case they should faint. If they go into a supermarket they panic if they have to wait at the checkout counter for any length of time. They often have difficulty travelling by bus or train because they fear they will not be able to get off in time if they feel faint. There is usually a clear distance from the house beyond which they will not go unless accompanied by someone else or a pet. They may also complain that they cannot tolerate being in closed spaces. They will try to organize their lives so that they avoid the feared situations. The woman may complain of a social phobia. She panics at the thought of meeting other people and will avoid this if possible. For example, if she and her husband are asked to go to dinner with friends, the woman will make excuses. She knows that if she goes she will feel self-conscious and worry that people are noticing every action. She will be scared that when she tries to eat or drink her hands will shake and this will be noticed. This could trigger panic and cause her to rush out of the room.

Occasionally, patients present with cancer phobias. Though they are free of disease and have been told so repeatedly they become terrified that they have cancer in the remaining breast or a recurrence. They often develop the habit of examining their breasts repeatedly to check for further cancer and persistently seek reassurance from doctors. Unfortunately, reassurance lasts only a short time and they soon consult again. This fear that they have cancer is usually accompanied by symptoms of generalized anxiety.

Sexual problems   Up to a third of patients who had an active and enjoyable sex life before surgery develop sexual problems (Morris et al, 1977; Maguire et al, 1978; Jamieson et al, 1978). They obtain much less, if any, enjoyment from sex, find it harder to achieve orgasm and may avoid intercourse altogether.

Body-image problems   As many as a fifth of women find it difficult to come to terms with the loss of a breast (Maguire et al, 1983). This may be because they cannot tolerate being less than physically whole. They may feel extremely self-conscious because they believe that other people can tell that they have had a mastectomy. This may cause marked social withdrawal, a change in the clothes they wear in order to conceal their shape, and the development of social phobias. Some women are devastated by the feeling that they are no longer attractive to others or feminine. Whatever the reason for the difficulty in adapting to the breast loss marked avoidance behaviour is common. The woman tries to prevent herself catching sight of her chest wall. She may do this by wearing a bra when in bed or by dressing and undressing in the dark. She may even change the height of mirrors or cover them up. This self-avoidance is usually accompanied by a refusal to allow her partner to see her naked.

Problems due to adjuvant chemotherapy

The use of cyclophosphamide, methotrexate and 5-fluorouracil in combination (CMF) leads to a greater psychiatric morbidity than can be accounted for by mastectomy alone (Maguire et al, 1980a; Cooper et al, 1979). The depression may be due to adverse effects like nausea, vomiting and hair loss or to a direct effect on the brain. The anxiety may also stem from adverse effects or from the development of a conditioned response. Any sight, sound, smell or thought which reminds them of chemotherapy causes them to feel nauseous and/or vomit reflexly (Morrow and Morrell, 1982). This can provoke panic and lead to phobic avoidance of treatment as well as generalized anxiety. CMF reduces oestrogen levels and elevates follicular stimulating and luteinizing hormones. So, premenopausal women undergo an artificial menopause and many patients experience a profound loss of libido. Difficulty in lubricating the vagina may cause dyspareunia. Sexual problems are, therefore, common in women given this treatment. Such changes in sexuality and other adverse effects like hair loss may intensify any body image problems.

Problems of recognition

In a surgical unit which was interested in the psychological welfare of women who undergo mastectomy, only a fifth of patients who developed psychological problems were recognized and offered help. Both patients and medical and nursing staff contribute to this hidden morbidity.

Patients

Women do not usually disclose that they have become anxious, depressed, or have developed sexual and body image problems, because they do not want to burden staff whom they see as busy and harassed. They also believe, albeit wrongly, that they are the only ones who are not coping and are afraid that if they admit this they will be seen as inadequate. They often also feel ashamed. They are aware that the doctors and nurses' priority is their physical wellbeing. They consider that it is not justifiable to mention other concerns. They may also believe their problems are inevitable and that nothing can be done about them.

Surgeons and nurses

Few surgeons, nurses, or general practitioners actively enquire how a patient is adjusting after mastectomy. In one study no patient was asked about her sex life after mastectomy. Similarly, patients are not usually asked about how they have been feeling in their spirits or how they have felt about losing a breast. Consequently, much of the morbidity remains hidden. Indeed, direct observation of surgeons and nurses interacting with breast cancer patients has found that they often, unwittingly, keep at an emotional distance from their patients. They selectively attend to cues about physical problems in preference to cues about psychological problems. They may manifestly ignore an obvious signal that the patient is distressed or try to deal with it by offering premature reassurance, that is, by saying 'it's all going to be all right' without having established what the patient is actually worried about. Sometimes, in a genuine bid to ease a patient's worry, they offer false reassurance by insisting that the patient will recover when they know already that this is unlikely. Other common distancing tactics include explaining away any emotional upset as normal. ('You are bound to be upset at this stage, everybody is but you will find you will soon get over it.') Alternatively, the doctor may simply switch the subject on to safer ground or try and jolly the patient out of it.

These distancing tactics prevent doctors and nurses getting close to patients and being confronted with even greater problems than are already posed by the breast cancer. Doctors and nurses fear that if they try to establish how a patient is suffering they will be faced with awkward questions, for example, about prognosis ('How long have I got?'), or the value of treatment ('Is it worth it?'). They are also afraid that they may unleash strong emotions like despair, anger and worry. They are not confident that they will be able to deal with such feelings, and they could be accused of upsetting patients. Moreover, it would take up too much time.

Doctors and nurses worry that they could get too involved and that this could be upsetting for them, if patients they liked were adversely affected by treatment or died. There is also the problem of identification. The patient might remind them of someone in their own life who has or could develop breast cancer. This could be emotionally draining. All these problems can be prevented by the use of distancing tactics, avoidance of appropriate questions, and the assumption, albeit false, that all patients who develop problems will disclose them. Consequently, some surgeons and nurses working with breast cancer patients genuinely believe that few women have any problems and find it hard to accept that a substantial proportion of women undergoing mastectomy develop serious problems. In practice, much can be done to improve the recognition and treatment of women who need psychological help.

Assessment
It is crucial that the surgeon is willing to enquire actively about the possibility of psychological problems. He can do this by the judicious use of questions which educate the patient that it is legitimate to disclose psychological matters.

Appropriate questions   It is useful to begin with an open question that directs attention to aspects other than physical health, for example: 'So far we've discussed how you have been getting on physically but how have you been in yourself since the operation?' Questions should also be addressed to specific areas like mood ('How have you been feeling in your spirits since you had your operation?'; 'Have you at any stage felt particularly low or miserable?'). If this reveals that the patient has become depressed, other questions should be asked to cover symptoms of depression like sleep disturbance, loss of energy or interest, irritability, and suicidal ideas. It is also important to screen for anxiety by asking: 'Have you felt especially worried or tense at any stage or in any particular situations?' In asking patients about sexual adjustment since surgery it is helpful to first check if this is acceptable by saying: 'Do you mind if I ask you about the physical aspect of your relationship with your husband since surgery?' and then ask: 'Have there been any problems?' The patient should be asked directly how she has reacted to losing a breast by enquiring: 'How have you felt about losing a breast?' or 'Has losing a breast affected you in any way?' Patients being treated with radiotherapy or chemotherapy should be asked routinely if it has been causing any problems or having particular side-effects. When adverse effects are evident, the patient's attitude towards further treatment should be elicited by saying, for example: 'In view of what you have said, how do you feel about continuing the treatment?' This should reveal if the patient has developed a conditioned response and begun to dread treatment so much that she has contemplated refusing it. The possibility that she may be suffering from anxiety, depression, body-image or sexual problems should be explored.

These questions do not take long but will reveal whether the patient has developed any psychological problems. The surgeon should then clarify the exact nature and extent of any problems in order to determine their severity. Once this has been done, whether in the ward or follow-up clinic, it is likely that on subsequent visits the patient will disclose spontaneously any problems which have developed.

Contributory factors
Once an anxiety state or depressive illness has been diagnosed, possible causes should be considered since this will influence management. The screening questions should have elicited whether it is due to fears of recurrence and/or the uncertainty of prognosis, an inability to adapt to the loss of a breast or adverse side-effects of chemotherapy (including conditioned responses). It is important to also consider that the development of mood disturbance may herald a recurrence of disease, metastatic spread, or be due to metabolic changes like hypercalcaemia. Steroids also provoke psychiatric disorder. When sexual problems arise, possible physical causes (like hormonal deficiencies due to chemotherapy, diabetes, recurrent disease, multiple sclerosis) and psychological causes (like anxiety, depression and body-image problems) should be considered.

In assessing body-image problems it is important to determine how much the patient tries to avoid catching sight of her chest wall and prevent her partner from looking. When a conditioned response to adjuvant chemotherapy has developed, the patient's attitude to further treatment should be explored as well as the possibility that this may have led her to become anxious, phobic or depressed.

Alternative methods of recognition

Both specialist and ward nurses (Faulkner and Maguire, 1984) can be taught to assess, recognize and refer for help the majority of those women who develop problems after mastectomy. This leads to a marked reduction in psychiatric morbidity (Maguire et al, 1980b). This requires practice with real patients, audiotape feedback of performance, and discussion with someone who is knowledgeable about interviewing and psychiatric assessment skills.

Prevention

There would be no need for surgeons to ask such questions if the psychological morbidity could be prevented by the provision of counselling before and after mastectomy. While adaptation to the breast loss and prosthesis can be facilitated, there is no firm evidence that the employment of specialist nurses or social workers prevents anxiety, depression or phobic states. However, counselling may have been ineffective because women were then undergoing a one-stage diagnosis, namely biopsy and frozen section – ?proceed to mastectomy. So, they were uncertain of the diagnosis when counselled preoperatively.

Treatment

Depressive illness

A depressive illness should be treated promptly with appropriate antidepressant treatment. New generation antidepressants like mianserin or dothiepin cause fewer adverse side-effects than the more established tricyclic antidepressants like amitriptyline and imipramine. This is important because patients who have been treated for cancer tend, wrongly, to attribute such side-effects to recurrence or spread of their disease, and compliance is also low. Whichever drug is chosen, it should be given in an effective dosage and continued for 4 to 6 months to forestall the risk of relapse. The rationale for treating depression should be explained on the basis that the stress of the illness or mastectomy has provoked a depressive illness which although understandable warrants treatment. It is also important to stress that it is not a tranquillizer and warn the patient that there could be side-effects like a dry mouth or drowsiness which should disappear as they adapt to the medication. It is helpful to indicate that these tablets take some time to work, otherwise patients may stop them because they believe they are ineffective. As the depression lifts it will become clear whether fears of recurrence or problems of adapting to breast loss remain.

Anxiety state   If the anxiety is overwhelming and the patient's ability to function impaired, an anxiolytic (like a benzodiazepine) should be used to alleviate it. If somatic aspects predominate, a beta-blocker (like propranolol) may be tried. If the woman is agitated a major tranquillizer (like thioridazine or chlorpromazine) should help.

If benzodiazepines are used for more than a few weeks, there is a risk that patients will become dependent on them. Major tranquillizers can cause unpleasant side-effects including extrapyramidal symptoms. So, once the drugs have begun to have an effect, it is helpful to teach patients how to manage their own anxiety.

Many patients suffering from anxiety benefit from being taught progressive muscular relaxation. They are shown how to systematically contract and relax major muscle groups and encouraged to relax (Janoun et al, 1982). Instructional audio-tapes can assist this. Once they have learned to relax they are asked to employ these techniques whenever they begin to feel anxious or are about to confront an anxiety-provoking situation. Patients can also be taught to summon up tranquil scenes to distract themselves and get rid of unwanted upsetting thoughts.

Those who develop agoraphobia, social phobias, or a disease phobia often benefit from desensitization. A hierarchy is first constructed of situations or thoughts which are most or least likely to provoke anxiety. She is taught to relax and asked to imagine an item low on the hierarchy, for example, 'When my breast feels prickly'. If she can imagine this situation without becoming anxious, she moves to the next item ('Pain in my breast') in the hierarchy. If a goal is not achieved, the patient is asked to relax again and reimagine the idea or situation.

Once an item has been managed in imagination, the patient can be encouraged to test it out in real life where appropriate. For example, once an agoraphobic patient is able to imagine walking from the front door to the gate without becoming anxious, she is advised to relax and then actually do this. It is possible to adopt a different approach (flooding) and start with items high on the hierarchy, but this is less popular with patients. The aim is to demonstrate, by preventing avoidance, that they can cope with a feared idea or situation.

Women with a cancer phobia who develop habits of repeated self-examination also benefit from being taught techniques of relaxation, distraction and thought-stopping. The therapist may also find response prevention useful. When the patient becomes anxious and wants to examine her remaining breast she is strongly discouraged.

Sexual problems   Most women respond well to the Masters and Johnson conjoint approach, where the woman and her partner are helped together (Masters and Johnson, 1970). This begins with a ban on sexual intercourse in order to lessen the woman's fear of it. The couple are then taught to find ways of pleasuring each other other than by genital contact. Once they have become confident in each other again they can proceed towards full intercourse. A major barrier to this can be a woman's inability to accept her breast loss and she will need desensitization or breast reconstruction before therapy can proceed.

Body-image problems
The use of progressive muscular relaxation and desensitization to looking at the chest wall, first in imagination and then in real life, is often effective in overcoming body-image problems. Once this is accomplished, the therapist may involve the husband or partner and encourage the woman to allow him to look again using relaxation and desensitization. In some women, the problems remain despite such help and a more cognitive approach may be useful. This involves challenging her assumptions that she is no longer attractive or of any use to anybody. She is actively encouraged to consider possible positive aspects of her situation. This might include the fact that the cancer was caught at an early stage. However, desensitization and cognitive therapy can fail to alleviate body-image problems and it is worth considering breast reconstruction. Women who want a reconstruction for themselves, rather than because pressure has been put on them by someone else, who are aware that they will get a cleavage rather than a breast as good as the original, and who are realistic about the possible complications of plastic surgery, respond well. Women who dislike the external prosthesis intensely because it slips around or because it reminds them of their cancer may also benefit.

Conditioned responses
When conditioning develops it is important to act promptly otherwise the patient may withdraw from treatment. Covering each major injection or infusion with an anxiolytic (like lorazepam), a major tranquillizer (like chlorpromazine) and/or an antiemetic may be sufficient. Teaching anxiety management techniques can also be effective (Burish and Lyles, 1981; Redd and Andrykowski, 1982; Morrow and Morrell, 1982). It is also important to treat any associated anxiety state or depressive illness with appropriate medication.

Cognitive therapy
When unreasonable fears of recurrence persist, cognitive therapy is useful (Goddard, 1982). It entails detailed examination of what is reasonable about her fears and what is unreasonable, as well as exploring what triggers these fears off and their consequences. Anxiety management techniques are also useful in conjunction with cognitive therapy to help the patient get to a point where she can combat her own fears and thoughts without the help of a therapist. This gives patients a strong sense that they can master their predicament. However, controlled trials

are still needed to determine the exact contribution made by antidepressants, anxiolytics and cognitive therapy to psychological recovery once a placebo effect has been allowed for.

Use of volunteers and self-help groups

When patients are experiencing problems it is useful to ask if they would like to talk with someone who has had a similar experience but overcome them. Such volunteers should be chosen carefully (Mantell, 1983). They should be able to listen, be flexible in their approach, avoid imposing their own experiences on the patient, and help the patient explore options rather than advise solutions. Otherwise, they may cause more harm than good.

Providing self-help groups are led by leaders who have a knowledge of group dynamics and who can help the group work constructively by allowing it to discuss real problems rather than become a psychotherapy group, they can be effective. They help women to feel less isolated after mastectomy and gain support from each other. Practical information and advice about available treatment options and what to do if problems arise can be discussed. Unfortunately, only one in ten women undergoing mastectomy are likely to make use of such groups.

Changing treatment policies

The adoption of simple tumour excision with breast conservation, or subcutaneous mastectomy, might reduce psychological morbidity. Any advantage might be offset by fears that some cancer remains and by problems caused by more intensive radiotherapy. Making a diagnosis in two stages should enhance adaptation. A woman can be told her diagnosis and then given time to consider and discuss her treatment options with whoever she chooses.

It has been claimed that immediate implantation at the time of surgery, and immediate or early reconstruction, reduces anxiety and depression (Schain et al, 1985), but it does not reduce sexual problems. It is possible that delayed implantation or reconstruction is preferable. The woman may be more realistic if she has experienced a period without her breast and is clear about her reasons for wanting this surgery.

The use of toxic adjuvant chemotherapy markedly increases morbidity which is something to bear in mind should the effect of such regimens be in doubt (Chapter 13). Tailoring information to what the woman wants to know and is ready to know and the provision of clear indicators of her progress should facilitate adjustment.

Controversies   • The identification of patients with psychological morbidity.
and Future   • The place of interventional therapy.
Developments

References

Burish, T.G. & Lyles, J.N. (1981) Effectiveness of relaxation training in reducing adverse reactions to cancer chemotherapy. *J. Behav. Med.*, *4*, 65–78.

Cooper, A.E., McArdle, C.S., Russell, A.R. & Smith, D.C. (1979) Psychiatric morbidity associated with adjuvant chemotherapy following mastectomy for breast cancer. *Br. J. Surg.*, *66*, 362.

Faulkner, A. & Maguire, P. (1984) Teaching ward nurses to monitor cancer patients. *Clin. Oncol.*, *10*, 383–389.

Goddard, A. (1982) Cognitive behaviour therapy and depression. *Br. J. Hosp. Med.*, *27*, 248–250.

Jamieson, K.R., Wellisch, D.K. & Pasnau, R.O. (1978) Psychosocial aspects of mastectomy: The woman's perspective. *Am. J. Psychiat.*, *135*, 432–436.

Janoun, L., Oppenheimer, C. & Gelder, M. (1982) A self-help treatment programme for anxiety-state patients. *Behav. Ther.*, *13*, 103–111.

Maguire, P. (1984a) Psychological reactions to breast cancer and its treatment. In: *Breast Cancer: Diagnosis and Management*, ed. Bonadonna, G. Bristol: John Wiley.

Maguire, P. (1984b) Counselling women with breast cancer. In: *Breast Cancer*, ed. Blamey, R.W. London: Update Publications.

Maguire, G.P., Lee, E.G., Bevington, D.J. et al (1978) Psychiatric problems in the first year after mastectomy. *Br. Med. J.*, *1*, 963–965.

Maguire, G.P., Tait, A., Brooke, M. et al (1980a) Psychiatric morbidity and physical toxicity associated with adjuvant chemotherapy after mastectomy. *Br. Med. J.*, *281*, 1179–1180.

Maguire, P., Tait, A., Brooke, M., Thomas, C. & Sellwood, R. (1980b) Effect of counselling on the psychiatric morbidity associated with mastectomy. *Br. Med. J.*, *281*, 1454–1456.

Maguire, P., Brooke, M., Tait, A., Thomas, C. & Sellwood, R. (1983) Effects of counselling on the physical disability and social recovery after mastectomy. *Clin. Oncol.*, *9*, 319, 324.

Mantell, J.E. (1983) Cancer patients' visitor programmes: a case for accountability. *J. Psychosoc. Oncol.*, *1*, 45–53.

Masters, W.E. & Johnson, V.E. (1970) *Human Sexual Inadequacy*. London: Bantam Books.

Morris, T. (1979) Psychological adjustment to mastectomy. *Cancer Treatment Rev.*, *6*, 41–61.

Morris, T., Greer, S.H. & White, P. (1977) Psychological and social adjustment to mastectomy. *Cancer*, *40*, 2381–2387.

Morrow, G.R. & Morrell, C. (1982) The antiemetic efficacy of behavioural treatment for cancer chemotherapy-induced anticipatory nausea and vomiting. *New Engl. J. Med.*, *307*, 1476–1480.

Redd, W.H. & Andrykowski, M.A. (1982) Behavioural intervention in cancer treatment:— controlling aversion reactions to chemotherapy. *J. Consult. Clin. Psychol.*, *50*, 1018–1029.

Schain, W.S., Wellisch, D.K., Pasnau, R.O. & Landsverk, J. (1985) The sooner the better: A study of psychological factors in women undergoing immediate versus delayed reconstruction. *Am. J. Psychiatry*, *142*, 1, 40–46.

16 Local Recurrence

Peter Blacklay

Local disease, in this chapter, describes recurrence of tumour in the skin flaps or remaining breast tissue, and is alternatively called flap recurrence. Often local disease is used to describe recurrence in the lymph nodes draining the breast tissue as well as recurrence in the flaps and scar; the two are separate in presentation, prognosis and therapy. Inclusion of lymph-node recurrence in reports of local disease obscures the incidence of flap recurrence. In data that make the distinction, flap recurrence occurs in between 2 and 20% of patients undergoing simple mastectomy. The highest incidence occurs in patients who undergo conservative surgery; this may reach 50% in subjects who have excision of the malignant lump alone.

Three types of flap recurrence commonly occur following mastectomy. Firstly, a spot recurrence may appear in the skin flaps or scar; this is a discrete circumspect nodule of malignant cells. Secondly, there are multiple-spot recurrences occurring synchronously (Fig. 16.1); again each is discrete, scattered over the scar and skin flaps. These may occur subsequent to a single spot recurrence. Thirdly, a field change may occur; this is entirely different to multiple recurrences in that it involves the whole area of skin flaps with a moist, thickened, somewhat eczematous appearance, and arises de novo (Fig. 16.2).

A third of all flap recurrences are discrete spots, a quarter are multiple spot recurrences, and the remainder are of the field-change type (Table 16.1).

The time of recurrence in the flaps is variable. Althoug' two-thirds of all flap recurrences have presented within the first two years following mastectomy, occasionally, skin flap recurrence has been reported 14 years after the initial mastectomy. The more aggressive field-change recurrence presents earlier than the other types.

The different types of flap recurrence arise following the removal of primary tumours with differing prognostic features. Those with subsequent spot or multiple-spot recurrence have a similar incidence of poor prognostic factors to those who do not develop any flap recurrence. Field change however occurs following the removal of an aggressive primary tumour which is poorly differentiated, has negative oestrogen status, and which has often spread to the draining lymph nodes.

Differing opinions as to the significance of flap recurrence have arisen in the past because of failure to recognize the

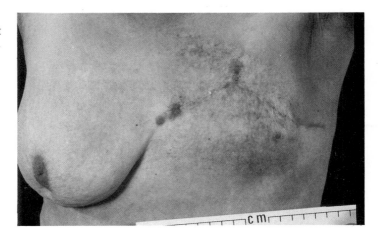

Figure 16.1
Multiple-spot
recurrence.

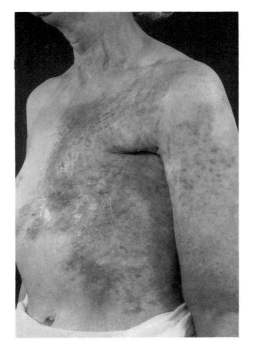

Figure 16.2
Field change—an
eczematous
appearance due to
infiltration of a wide
area of skin with
tumour.

different types that occur. In fact, although each type has a
significantly worse prognosis than those patients without flap
recurrence, there is a rank order from single spot, through
multiple spot, to field change. Just over one-third of those with
single spots and only 5% of those with field change survive five
years from mastectomy. Freedom from distant metastases follows
a similar pattern, with all those in the field-change group

Type of flap recurrence	No.	Treatment	Lasting control (or until death)
Single spot	30	Excision	22
Multiple spot after single spot	8	Radiotherapy	8
Multiple spot de novo	8	Radiotherapy	8
Field change	28	Radiotherapy	9

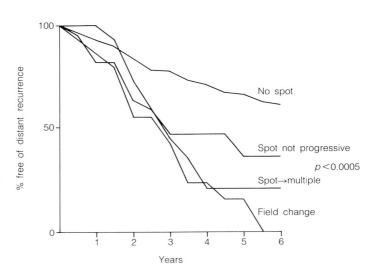

developing symptomatic distant metastases by five years (Fig. 16.3).

Treatment of local recurrence

Diagnosis is easily made by biopsy which proves the nature of the tissue and the clinical appearance then categorizes the flap recurrence. This is important for two reasons, firstly, it gives an insight into prognosis, and, secondly, it directs therapy.

Local therapy can be used in the majority of cases. The spot recurrence is treated by diagnostic excision biopsy. Local anaesthetic is used to infiltrate the area, the nodule is excised with 2 mm of normal tissue surrounding the recurrence, and primary closure is gained. This can be repeated with any subsequent discrete nodules, so long as there is adequate skin mobility.

Multiple-spot recurrences are excluded from local excision because skin closure would not be possible. Diagnosis is made by excision biopsy of one of the nodules and radiotherapy is used to gain control.

Field change may be treated by radiotherapy but, as observed above, it is in fact the herald of the appearance of distant metastases. Systemic therapy may be more appropriate but, even here, it is unlikely to succeed because of the aggressive nature of the type of tumour which gives field change.

The first-line local therapy, of excision or radiotherapy, to the spot or multiple-spot recurrences gains complete control in 80% (Table 16.1). Field change has a poor response to first-line therapy, with only one-third gaining complete control with radiotherapy.

Controversies and Future Developments

• The identification of patients likely to suffer flap recurrence and the place of prophylactic local and systemic therapies in these patients.

17 Axillary Recurrence

Michael Williams

In Halsted's radical operation for breast cancer, removal of subpectoral and axillary lymphatic tissue is performed as well as mastectomy. The operation was devised nearly a century ago and soon after this time the theory was first enunciated that cancer spreads as a solid core of tissue along lymphatics to regional lymph nodes, which are then the invariable source of distant metastasis. It was envisaged that early irradiation of these nodes along with the primary tumour would be curative. The incidence of recurrence in the axilla and in the skin flap fashioned after mastectomy is less after a radical than after a limited resection, but survival is not significantly improved and supraradical mastectomy involving the removal of more of the adjacent lymphatic tissue, including supraclavicular and internal mammary nodes, confers no added survival benefit.

Radiotherapy was introduced in the management of breast cancer around the second decade of the 20th century and was soon found to be an effective addition to surgery for the control of cancer spreading locally beyond the primary site. It has been shown that irradiation after radical mastectomy can further reduce the incidence of both local and regional recurrence. In an American trial, the National Surgical Adjuvant Breast Project (Fisher et al, 1975) of 1103 patients who had undergone radical mastectomy, 470 were randomly selected to receive postoperative radiotherapy. The remainder, serving as a control group, received no radiotherapy. Despite 50% of the control group also receiving adjuvant systemic treatment, of the patients treated with radiotherapy 0.6% developed regional recurrence during the five year observation period compared with 6% in the control group, a small but significant reduction. No improvement in survival was noted.

Other trials have compared the results of radical surgery with those of simple mastectomy combined with radiotherapy and have shown no advantage in terms of survival or in a reduction in the incidence of local recurrence (Host and Brennhoyd, 1977). In the United Kingdom, therefore, radical surgery has largely been replaced by simple mastectomy. There has been continuing discussion concerning whether such surgery should be accompanied by radiotherapy.

Prophylactic treatment of regional nodes
The Cancer Research Campaign reported the findings in a series of 2243 patients treated with simple mastectomy, either alone or

combined with postoperative radiotherapy. A watch policy was adopted whereby patients not treated at the time of mastectomy received radiotherapy at the presentation of locally recurrent disease. Those patients receiving prophylactic radiotherapy showed a markedly lower incidence of recurrent local or axillary disease (11% as compared with 30% at five years), but survival over 10 years was not improved. The probability of developing local or regional recurrence can thus be reduced to one-third by immediate radiotherapy after simple mastectomy. When radiotherapy is given routinely, those patients with biologically favourable tumours who would not develop locally recurrent disease will have been treated unnecessarily and there is no evidence that delaying treatment until patients with aggressive tumours become symptomatic either compromises survival or reduces the chance of disease control once this occurs.

In many centres involvement of axillary nodes at the time of mastectomy is considered an indication for radiotherapy which is intended to prolong the disease-free interval. Although lymph-node staging correlates well with survival and postoperative axillary recurrence, some patients found to have involvement of axillary nodes do not develop symptomatic axillary disease and others with nodal enlargement die of disseminated disease without symptomatic reasons for local treatment. The appearance of involved nodes in the axilla is often the harbinger of distant metastasis. In one series (Chu et al, 1976) clinical evidence of dissemination followed after an average interval of only 22 months. In our series of those patients developing symptomatic local or regional disease within 48 months of presentation only 20% were alive at 72 months (Fig. 17.1).

The prediction of regional recurrence
Certain factors recordable at the time of mastectomy have been studied in an attempt to facilitate the identification of patients

Figure 17.1 Survival after locoregional recurrence following mastectomy for operable primary breast cancer.

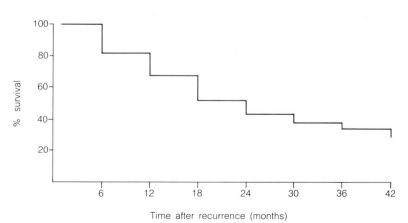

Time after recurrence (months)

Table 17.1
Locoregional recur-
rence at 48 months
from mastectomy:
lymph node stage and
tumour grade.

	Histological grade		
	I	II	III
Lymph node-negative			
Total	46	77	113
Locoregional recurrence at 48 months	6	7	24
% chance of recurrence	13	9	21
Lymph node-positive			
Total	25	77	101
Locoregional recurrence at 48 months	1	19	48
% chance of recurrence	4	25	48

most likely to develop symptomatic local or regional recurrence. Of these factors in one enquiry only the grade of the primary tumour and the lymph node status were of independent discriminatory value. Four hundred and thirty-nine patients were kept under surveillance in Nottingham for a minimum of four years with a maximum follow-up of ten years. Eighty per cent of local or regional recurrences occurring over the total study period presented within four years from mastectomy.

In this study prophylactic radiotherapy had not been employed and all patients receiving treatment for locally recurrent disease did so for symptomatic reasons. Surgical excisions of mastectomy flap recurrences or symptomatic axillary nodes were performed initially where indicated, resorting to radiotherapy when minor surgery was not possible. By employing this regimen, 119 patients required local treatments over the 10 years of follow-up. When combining prognostic factors (Grade III tumours, lymph node-positive at mastectomy) a group which contained only 23% of all patients was identified in which more than 40% of symptomatic local and regional recurrences occurred (Table 17.1).

The purpose of prophylactic radiotherapy after simple mastectomy is to reduce the incidence of symptomatic local recurrence. It should therefore be reserved for those patients most likely to require treatment, thus reducing cost and postradiotherapy complications. The benefit of adjuvant radiotherapy for the patient identified as being at risk is solely the psychological advantage of a prolongation in disease-free interval. Survival is not improved and delayed radiotherapy usually controls any local recurrence which has arisen (Cancer Research Campaign Working Party, 1980).

Radiotherapy after simple mastectomy is usually well tolerated. After radical mastectomy or any procedure involving extensive exploration and dissection in the axilla, its complications can be serious and are considered prohibitive by many.

Lymphoedema is refractory to treatment and when there is gross involvement of the arm, pain and discomfort is associated with severe impairment of function.

Presentation of regional recurrence

Involvement of lymph nodes may be discovered routinely, they may be asymptomatic, or, on the other hand, the patient may present with pain in the axilla or pain referred along the arm. The finding of a swelling in the axilla is often the cause of anxiety, itself then an indication for treatment. An axillary mass when grossly enlarged can cause lymphatic and venous obstruction, resulting in lymphoedema and swelling of the arm. Further disease progression often due to neglect can lead to fungation and ulceration with secondary infection.

Treatment of regional recurrence

Axillary lymph nodes which are small and freely mobile can usually be excised without difficulty and there are no postoperative complications. When disease recurs in the axilla after previous surgical excision, radiotherapy may gain control. In one series of patients with local or regional recurrence after mastectomy, partial or complete response to radiotherapy was observed in 91% of 215 patients (Chu et al, 1976). When nodes are clinically inoperable, due for example to involvement of large vessels and nerves, radiotherapy is the initial treatment of choice. Progression despite surgery or radiotherapy is an indication for systemic hormone treatment, as are the presence of distant metastases. In many patients systemic therapy can be avoided or deferred by partial resection of the axillary mass followed by a course of radiotherapy. When patients with distant metastases respond to systemic treatment, both local and distant disease is controlled simultaneously. For the non-responders palliative radiotherapy may again be indicated.

Supervoltage radiotherapeutic techniques introduced in the 1950s have replaced orthovoltage treatment, with a consequent dramatic reduction in the incidence and severity of complications. Supervoltage therapy allows deep penetration into tumour tissue, causing less damage to the skin and other superficial structures. Skin desquamation and pain, however, are still common after radical radiotherapy and the high risk of skin necrosis precludes its repeated use in the same site. Surgical excision, therefore, remains the treatment of choice with radiotherapy being given when surgery is inappropriate.

Rarely, in patients who do not have distant metastases, local disease progresses inexorably despite surgery, radiotherapy and endocrine treatment. Radical local 'toilet' surgery can sometimes reduce the appalling symptoms due to extensive fungation or ulceration, although deciding on management can be difficult. Large defects resulting from extensive surgery may be covered by the use of omental flaps. Cytotoxic drug treatment is of some value as palliation when patients with extensive localized recurrent disease are unresponsive to other measures, but at this advanced stage the morbidity of such aggressive treatment is considerable.

Lymphoedema

After fungation and ulceration, lymphoedema of the arm is probably the most distressing complication of axillary recurrent disease (Chapter 10). Sometimes, regrettably, it is iatrogenic, the direct result of extensive surgery in the axilla followed by radiotherapy. In a recent study clinical lymphoedema was found in 51% of patients 2–4 months after radical mastectomy as compared with 19% after a modified procedure. The highest rate was observed (64%) in patients who had received both radical surgery and postoperative radiotherapy (Brismar and Ljungdahl, 1983).

Aggressive local disease requiring surgical excision and radiotherapy as a secondary procedure can also compromise lymphatic drainage to a degree sufficient to cause clinical lymphoedema. The limb may be rendered useless and when changes are gross the patient may experience severe pain often of a bursting nature. The treatment of lymphoedema is unsatisfactory. Pneumatic compression of the upper limb with an inflatable cuff may produce some symptomatic relief but the procedure may have to be repeated at frequent intervals. Elevation of the limb at night can also help to reduce swelling. Surgery should be avoided; it often results in deterioration and impairment of postoperative wound healing is an added risk.

Summary

Present evidence suggests that axillary recurrent disease is best managed overall by adopting a watch policy in preference to a policy of routine prophylactic radiotherapy at the time of simple mastectomy. Our present policy is to treat only nodes which become enlarged and give rise to symptoms (see above). If prophylactic treatment is preferred it should be offered only to those patients at high risk of requiring subsequent local treatment and these can be identified by a combination of tumour grade and lymph-node stage at the time of mastectomy. The complications of radiotherapy are sometimes severe and routine irradiation is best avoided in patients not at high risk of requiring this treatment.

Controversies and Future Developments

- The identification of patients likely to suffer symptomatic axillary recurrence and their prophylactic treatment.

References

Brismar, B. & Ljungdahl, I. (1983) Postoperative lymphoedema after treatment of breast cancer. *Acta Chir. Scand.*, *149*, 687–689.

Cancer Research Campaign Working Party (1980) Cancer Research Campaign (King's /Cambridge) trial for early breast cancer. *Lancet, ii,* 55–60.

Chu, F.C., Lin, F.J., Kim, J.H. et al (1976) Locally recurrent carcinoma of the breast. Results of radiation therapy. *Cancer, 37,* 2677–2681.

Fisher, B., Slack, N., Katrych, D. & Wolmark, N. (1975) Ten-year follow-up results of patients with carcinoma of the breast in a co-operative clinical trial evaluating surgical adjuvant chemotherapy. *Surg. Gynecol. Obstet., 140,* 528–534.

Halsted, W.S. (1907) Results of radical operations for the cure of carcinoma of the breast. *Ann. Surg., 46,* 1–19.

Host, H. & Brennhovd, I.O. (1977) The effect of post operative radiotherapy in breast cancer. *Int. J. Radiot. Oncol. Bio. Phys., 2,* 1061–1067.

18 Care of the Patient in Follow-up and Introduction to Systemic Therapy of Metastatic Spread

Roger Blamey

This chapter introduces the next few chapters in which the options available for the systemic therapy of metastatic spread are discussed.

Factors measured at the time of diagnosis of a primary breast cancer can be used to give a good index of those patients who have distant metastases which will one day present and affect the chance of five and ten year survival. However, there is no proven advantage, in terms of survival, in implementing treatment directed against the distant spread at the time of diagnosis over reserving any treatment until the metastases become clinically apparent (Chapter 13).

After treatment of the primary disease there is an apparent 'tumour-free interval' until the patient presents with symptoms of metastatic spread: these are most commonly bone pain, dyspnoea due to pleural effusion or to lung infiltration, tiredness, and marked anorexia due to liver metastases or a variety of symptoms from CNS spread. Added to or separate from these may be regional lymph-node enlargement or local skin flap recurrences.

Follow-up in the disease-free interval
Regular follow-up during the tumour-free interval is necessary in two respects—to investigate symptoms which may be due to metastases, and to keep an eye on the opposite breast.

Dealing first with the latter, women with breast cancer have an increased risk of developing cancer of the opposite breast: the risk is around 1–2% per annum and this risk is maintained and does not fall off with the years (Chaudray et al, 1984). Therefore, regular mammographic checks of the opposite breast would seem necessary; however, this would impose a considerable load on hospital X-ray departments. There is little point in screening the opposite breast of a woman who is going to die from metastases from her first breast cancer. Our recommendation is to use prognostic indices (Haybittle et al, 1982) to select the group of women likely to do well following treatment of their breast cancer; this group only should have biennial mammography included in their follow-up.

The investigation of symptoms from metastatic spread in breast cancer may seem straightforward; however, very often the root of these symptoms may be unrecognized for several months by the patient's practitioner. This is particularly so in several syndromes: breathlessness from pulmonary carcinomatous lymphagitis (which is often put down to cardiac failure since the X-ray may be difficult to interpret); hypercalcaemia; CNS metastases. Even symptoms of bone pain or nerve root irritation may be insufficiently investigated. Therefore, in our clinic, we prefer to maintain regular checks by the breast cancer team in follow-up.

General principles of treatment of metastases

Once symptoms from metastases are recognized and correctly diagnosed, then therapy is instituted. In every case two simultaneous lines are indicated: systemic therapy and 'local therapy'. By local therapy, I mean therapy directed to the specific symptom: irradiation of painful bone or of brain metastases, treatment of hypercalcaemia, drainage of pleural or pericardial effusion, administration of dexamethazone for CNS symptoms, surgical decompression of the spinal cord, fixation of bone fractures, general treatment of dyspnoea.

Since survival from the time of diagnosis of metastatic spread is heavily dependent upon whether, and how well, the patient responds to endocrine therapy (Fig. 18.1), and since, in general, response to chemotherapy is poor in breast cancer, we first pursue endocrine therapy.

As first-line endocrine therapy the postmenopausal patient receives tamoxifen (Nolvadex, ICI), a treatment virtually with-

Figure 18.1
Survival from start of treatment for secondary breast cancer—patients with objective response to endocrine therapy versus non-responders.

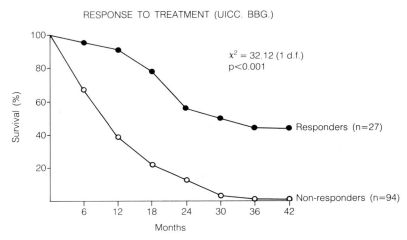

RESPONSE TO TREATMENT (UICC. BBG.)

$x^2 = 32.12$ (1 d.f.)
$p < 0.001$

Responders (n=27)

Non-responders (n=94)

Survival (%)

Months

out side-effects; the premenopausal woman until recently has undergone oophorectomy (although there are now options which do not require operative treatment—see Chapter 19).

If the tumour shows objective response to first-line hormone therapy, then when it relapses from control a second-line hormone therapy is instituted. There are a number of alternatives. Clinical trials comparing different forms of therapy at this stage of disease are difficult to carry out. Without these it would seem that there is little advantage to one treatment over any other in terms of response rate and duration. Therefore, the treatment used is based on assessment of the side-effects. As examples, two such therapies are discussed in Chapters 20 and 21 and their complications compared.

Another operative alternative is hypophysectomy, although in terms of operative technique and length of operation, postoperative discomfort and length of hospital stay, this operation has no clear advantage over adrenalectomy. Hypophyseal implantation with ^{90}Yt is simple once learnt, with a very short operative time and little side-effect. It does carry the chance of considerable technical morbidity in the learning phase for the individual surgeon or radiotherapist, in the form of damage to the optic chiasma or to the nerves controlling eye movements. Hypophyseal removal on ablation requires long-term corticosteroid replacement plus vasopressin snuff for diabetes insipidus.

Our present preference in second-line hormone treatment is for high dose progesterone treatment: Megace (Bristol-Myers). We give 320 mg orally per day—side-effects are as for glucocorticords, with weight gain pronounced. However, there is often a useful euphoric effect. Androgens are used in some centres but have masculinizing side-effects in addition to the cortisone effect.

If tumour does not respond to first-line hormone therapy then the chance of response to second-line is poor, and cytotoxic chemotherapy may be introduced. Chemotherapeutic regimes often have unpleasant side-effects (Chapter 22) and where response occurs it is usually short-lived. The patient's life expectancy is short, and after any remission the metastases will again progress and give symptoms. Therefore the individual circumstances must be considered before taking the decision to give cytotoxic therapy. Palliation of breathlessness in pulmonary lymphangitis and of local or regional disease which has failed to respond to other measures, are the most worthwhile for treatment. On the other hand, liver metastases, and particularly CNS metastases, are not usually treated with cytotoxics. There is no indication for aggressive cytotoxic therapy and our present preference is for low dose single-agent chemotherapy used for three months, continued if a response is seen, with a switch to another agent if there is progression of disease.

Whatever the decision on systemic therapy by an individual unit, a clear overall policy should be made. The multiplicity of

Figure 18.2
General plan of systemic therapies in patients with secondary breast cancer.

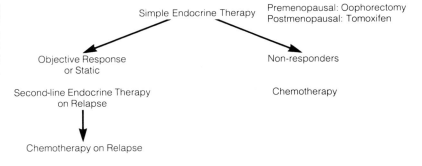

agents and the diverse reports on them would make management extremely confused without such a plan. The plan on our unit presented above is summarized in Fig. 18.2.

Controversies and Future Developments

- The place of predictive factors for response in selecting patients for endocrine therapy.
- Which patients should receive second-line hormone therapy and selection of appropriate therapy.
- The selection of some patients for early chemotherapy.
- Better prediction for endocrine therapy (monoclonal antibody to ER).
- Prediction of response to chemotherapy.
- Laboratory-based measurement of response to therapy.

References

Chaudray, M.A., Millis, R.R., Hoskins, E.O.L. et al (1984) Bilateral primary breast cancer: a prospective study of disease incidence. *Br. J. Surg.*, *71*, 711–714.

Haybittle, J.L., Blamey, R.W., Elston, C.W. et al (1982) A prognostic index in primary breast cancer. *Br. J. Cancer*, *45*, 361–366.

19 The Premenopausal Woman

Michael Williams and Robert Nicholson

It has long been known that hormonal factors may have a profound influence on the growth characteristics of advanced breast cancer. Schinzinger in 1899 first suggested that surgical castration (oophorectomy) could be used as a therapeutic manoeuvre in the desperate attempt to slow the progression of advanced disease. Beatson in 1896 reported the first clinical responses to this form of treatment in inoperable cases. His findings were soon confirmed by Boyd in 1900 who claimed 'improvement' in 37% of 46 premenopausal patients treated in this way. Patients who responded survived for 16.5 months compared to an average survival of 5 months for the remainder.

Decourmelles in 1922 suggested that the induction of an artificial menopause by irradiation was a realistic alternative to surgical oophorectomy and in 1936 Dresser reported an improvement in 30% of a series of patients with bone metastases treated in this way.

Later investigators have assessed the rate of regression after surgical oophorectomy, comparing it with that achieved by ovarian irradiation, and have found that surgery, by producing a prompt fall in circulating oestrogens, is more rapidly effective. This is an advantage of particular importance to patients with rapidly progressing disease. The overall response rates, however, to both forms of treatment are the same and it is generally agreed that ovarian ablation whether achieved by surgery or by irradiation is effective in the treatment of advanced breast cancer.

It is clear that between one-third and two-thirds of patients undergoing therapeutic ablation of the ovaries will show signs of a response to treatment which is associated with a prolongation of survival. This prolongation of survival cannot necessarily be attributed entirely to endocrine ablation since patients who respond to treatment may well be a selected group, whose tumours are biologically associated with a relatively prolonged survival despite treatment.

Response to oophorectomy is almost completely confined to patients who are premenopausal at the presentation of disseminated disease. Such patients will show symptomatic improvement with regression of local and disseminated disease. When bone metastases are present, a reduction in bone pain is often associated with sclerosis of lytic metastases demonstrated radio-logically. The introduction of major endocrine ablation in the treatment of breast cancer followed the realization that other endocrine glands can take over the production of hormones formerly released by the ovaries. Patients who have earlier responded to oophorectomy are more likely than non-responders to benefit from major endocrine ablation, in one series 54% compared with 9.5% (Stewart, 1970).

Prediction of response to oophorectomy

The use of surgical oophorectomy is confined to premenopausal patients with advanced breast cancer. This is, of course, logical since ovarian function is physiologically diminishing over this period and any effects of further ablative procedures are reduced. Some reports claim significant but reduced response rates in patients immediately postmenopausal, but caution must be taken when interpreting these results since studies use different criteria to define the natural menopause.

Stewart reviewed a large series of patients undergoing ovarian ablation for advanced disease and found that one-third of patients within two years of their last menstrual period res-ponded to treatment as compared to only 5% of those two to five years from this time. In the same series an improved remission

Figure 19.1
Quantitative ER concentrations in the primary tumour and subsequent response to endocrine therapy.

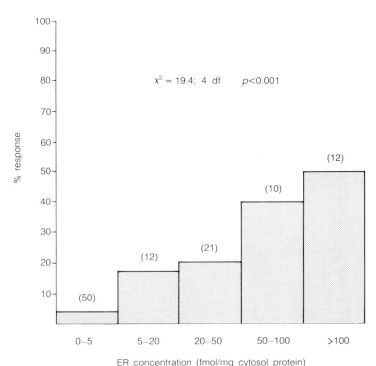

ER concentration (fmol/mg cytosol protein)

rate was achieved in those patients with generalized disease compared with those with local disease only. Other studies have reported lower response rates in bone metastases compared to those seen in soft-tissue sites. This in part may be due to the greater difficulty in assessing responses in metastatic bone lesions. Response rates in liver are uniformly low in all reported series.

The discovery of receptor proteins in the cytosolic fraction of tumour cells was made by Jenson in 1971. Demonstrating the presence of these proteins is helpful in predicting the response of advanced disease to endocrine ablation. Assays for oestrogen and progesterone receptor can be performed either on the primary tumour or on any accessible secondary deposit. The response rate to oophorectomy reported for tumours containing the oestrogen receptor has ranged from 40%–60%, compared with less than 10% in patients with oestrogen receptor-negative tumours.

Quantitative oestrogen receptor assays (Fig. 19.1) and the progesterone receptor assay can further improve the value of these investigations in defining patients most likely to respond to endocrine manipulation. On the other hand, it must be acknowledged that while the absence of measureable receptors correlates closely with treatment failure, the predictive accuracy of the presence of receptors is only around 50%.

The use of tamoxifen in premenopausal advanced breast cancer

Tamoxifen is a synthetic non-steroidal compound with antioestrogen activity. It has a structure similar to diethyl stilboestrol and was introduced by ICI in 1970 to palliate postmenopausal patients with advanced breast cancer. Prior to this time such patients had been treated with oestrogens or androgens. The main advantage that this new therapy had over previously accepted treatments lay not so much in any increase in response rate but more in its lack of toxicity. The cardiovascular side-effects of oestrogens are well documented and the weight gain and virilization associated with androgenic therapies were a disadvantage when these treatments were employed.

Circulating oestrogens are freely absorbed into all cells. Certain tissues (e.g. the uterus and breast) possess oestrogen

Table 19.1
Response to tamoxifen in postmenopausal patients.

	Patients	*Response*
Cole	129	28 (22%)
Ward	68	28 (38%)
Brewin	103	28 (27%)
Westerberg	89	38 (43%)
Ribeiro	141	36 (25%)

receptors in the cytoplasm of their cells which increase the affinity for oestrogens and are necessary for oestrogen-induced tissue growth.

Tamoxifen, like oestrogens, is also able to bind to oestrogen receptor proteins, but produces a receptor complex which is unable to stimulate or maintain growth. When administered clinically, tamoxifen reaches tumour tissue concentrations far in excess of those observed for oestrogens and thereby competes out the normal binding of these hormones to tumour oestrogen receptor proteins. This results in a cessation of tumour growth in sensitive lesions and may promote tumour remissions.

Clinical   The effectiveness of tamoxifen in the treatment of patients with
studies   advanced breast cancer presenting after the menopause is acknowledged; about one-third are likely to respond (Table 19.1). Encouraged also by an understanding of its pharmacological action, the value of treatment with tamoxifen before the menopause has recently been examined. Response rates have compared favourably with those after ovarian ablation; a third of patients are likely to respond and the prediction of a response is helped by oestrogen receptor assays.

Pritchard et al (1980) evaluated tamoxifen in 42 premenopausal patients. All patients had either had a menstrual period within six months of entry into the trial or were under 50 years of age and had undergone previous hysterectomy with conservation of ovarian tissue. None had undergone bilateral oophorectomy or received previous endocrine therapy. Thirty-six patients were prescribed tamoxifen, 40 mg daily. In 2 patients the dosage of tamoxifen was escalated at 11 and 12 weeks in unsuccessful attempts to attain remission. For those patients who responded or who did not appear to deteriorate, treatment was continued; the remainder underwent surgical or irradiation ovarian ablation. Three patients were claimed to have shown complete response to tamoxifen, 10 patients partial response (i.e. more than 50% reduction in tumour size) and in 4 patients the disease remained stable. The overall complete and partial response rate therefore was 32%.

In assessing the predictive value of receptor assays, one patient with a negative assay for oestrogen or progesterone receptors remained stable; 8 failed to respond. In contrast, 8 of 18 patients with a positive assay for oestrogen or progesterone receptors responded or remained stable on treatment. Of the 25 patients who failed to respond to tamoxifen, 13 later underwent ovarian ablation without benefit. Of the patients who responded to tamoxifen, 9 later developed progressive disease, 8 of these underwent ovarian ablation, only 1 failed to respond.

It would appear therefore that the steroid receptor status of the primary tumour is useful in predicting the response to tamoxifen in patients treated before the menopause; furthermore, this response is a good indicator of a later response to oophorectomy.

Figure 19.2a,b
UK multicentre trial
comparing
oophorectomy with
tamoxifen in first-line
treatment for
advanced breast
cancer in
premenopausal
women. Despite low
patient numbers
(*n*=122) the curves
are unlikely to cross
over with time (note
that the proportion
with events is high).

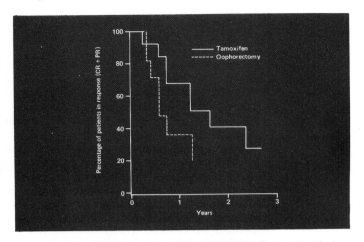

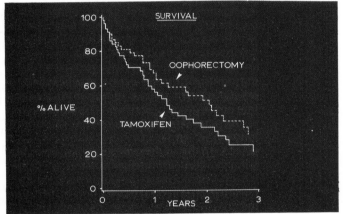

Similar findings have been reported by Wada et al (1981) from Japan, and a recent five-centre controlled trial in the UK, to which the Nottingham Breast clinic contributed, has shown no difference in response or survival in patients treated by tamoxifen as compared with oophorectomy (Fig. 19.2).

Summary   Recent reports have confirmed the effectiveness of tamoxifen as a treatment for advanced breast cancer presenting before the menopause. A favourable response can be anticipated in a third of the patients, results similar to those after oophorectomy. A response to tamoxifen is also a predictor of a later response to ovarian ablation, but its precise role in treatment will become clear when further information from randomized trials becomes available. Side-effects are few. They include menstrual cessation or irregularities, flushes, nausea, vomiting and headache. In patients with bone metastases, tumour flare may cause transient hypercalcaemia, and jaundice has also been reported as a rare complication in postmenopausal patients.

The use of LH/RH agonists in advanced premenopausal breast cancer

Luteinizing hormone-releasing hormone (LH-RH) is produced by the hypothalamus and controls the pituitary gland release of follicle stimulating hormone (FSH) and luteinizing hormone (LH) throughout the menstrual cycle. For normal function the pituitary gland is stimulated by pulses of LH-RH, producing pulsatile secretion of the gonadotrophins and maintaining cyclical gonadal function. Treatment of animals or patients with hyperphysiological concentrations of LH-RH agonists overrides the normal pattern of LH-RH release and leads to a fall in circulating levels of LH and FSH and a withdrawal of their support for gonadal activity (Nicholson et al, 1979). It was the potential beneficial effects of such actions on hormone-dependent breast cancer that has lead to recent clinical trials using these agents in premenopausal advanced breast cancer.

The potential value of LH-RH agonists in the treatment of advanced breast cancer has recently been examined. Twenty-seven premenopausal patients with recurrent or locally advanced breast cancer were treated with Zoladex (ICI 118630) after informed consent had been obtained. None had received prior treatment for advanced disease. The drug was administered subcutaneously, 500–1000 μg daily, soon after the diagnosis of inoperable or metastatic disease had been established and at a time inconstantly related to the menstrual cycle.

Zoladex is now available in a slow-release preparation that will require injection only once per month.

Endocrine response

Circulating levels of luteinizing hormone, follicle stimulating hormone, oestradiol and progesterone were measured throughout treatment. Clinical response was closely monitored and surgical oophorectomy was performed at the first evidence of disease progression. Regardless of the phase of the menstrual cycle at the commencement of treatment, consistent changes were found in LH and FSH levels. A prompt increase followed the first injection of Zoladex, levels falling to basal values during the same or subsequent menstrual cycle. The early rise in circulating LH and FSH was associated with a small inconsistent rise in oestradiol and progesterone. This was noted especially when treatment was started in the early follicular phase of the menstrual cycle. Plasma progesterone then returned to normal basal values, thereafter remaining low, indicating that ovulation and formation of an active corpus luteum had been inhibited. Plasma oestradiol fell towards the onset of the next menstrual cycle, remaining low for the remainder of the study, during which time no further menstrual activity was observed (Fig. 19.3). When treatment was started in mid-cycle or during the luteal (later)

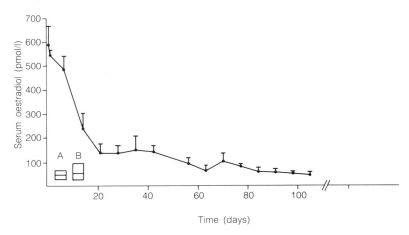

Figure 19.3
LH-RH agonist
(Zoladex). Long-term
effects on plasma
oestradiol in patients
with advanced breast
cancer (mean+SEM).
A=postmenopausal;
B=oophorectomized.

phase of the menstrual cycle, circulating levels of oestradiol and progesterone were unaltered until the following cycle. A fall in circulating oestradiol was then observed, progesterone no longer being detectable. On continuing treatment, circulating oestrogens were further suppressed and secondary amenorrhoea became established in all patients. The immediate effect of Zoladex on pituitary function was examined and also the effects of treatment continued for several weeks (i.e. 38–82 days).

After the first injection there was a marked rise in the plasma FSH and LH concentrations. After prolonged treatment no such elevation was noted, the pituitary gland having become desensitized. In three patients treated for almost a year circulating oestradiol and progesterone have remained low.

Clinical response

Assessment of a response to Zoladex was made using UICC criteria with the stipulation that any response should be of at least six months' duration.

Zoladex has been administered to 27 patients; of these 21 are assessable on these criteria.

The predominant sites of metastases are shown in Table 19.2. The initial assessment, prior to commencing treatment, included documentation and photography of all local disease. A skeletal survey was performed on all patients and isotope hepatic and bone scans if clinically indicated.

All patients tolerated treatment well without unpredictable side-effects. Perimenopausal symptoms, hot flushes and/or nausea, were observed in 11 patients undergoing therapy, and cessation of normal menstruation on long-term treatment occurred in all patients. A partial response to Zoladex was observed in 4 patients, in 1 patient disease remained stable and in the remaining 16 disease progressed. In all patients surgical oophorectomy was performed on disease progression. A subsequent response to oophorectomy was documented in 4 patients

Table 19.2
Sites of metastases
pretreatment with
Zoladex.

Local only	6	Bone and lung	5
Bone only	5	Bone and local	2
Lung only	2	Bone, lung, liver	1

while disease remained static at six months in 2 patients. No objective response to treatment occurred in the remaining 10 patients undergoing surgical oophorectomy. The overall response rate to Zoladex in this series was therefore 19%.

Other studies

The effectiveness of LH-RH agonists in the treatment of advanced breast cancer has been confirmed in a further study (Klijn, 1984). The agonist buserelin (Hoe-766) was given to 17 patients presenting before the menopause. Twelve received buserelin alone as initial treatment and in 5 it was combined with tamoxifen. In 9 of the 12 patients initially prescribed buserelin alone, tamoxifen was later added either because of a rise in plasma oestradiol or because of clinical progression. Buserelin was first administered parenterally; treatment was then continued by intranasal insufflation.

Four of the 12 patients initially prescribed buserelin alone responded, 2 partially, and in 2 a complete response occurred. In 4 patients disease remained static. A further 2 patients in this group responded partially after the addition of tamoxifen and in all patients anovulation and suppression of progesterone had occurred. Transient peaks of oestradiol were, however, observed in 60% of patients treated with buserelin alone. In 2 of the group of patients initially treated with buserelin alone a secondary rise in plasma oestradiol was effectively suppressed by tamoxifen. In 3 others recurrent plasma peaks of oestradiol and reappearance of progesterone secretion occurred after the addition of tamoxifen. In 1 patient plasma oestradiol was exceptionally high but tumour progression did not take place.

Of the 5 patients treated throughout with buserelin and tamoxifen, 2 responded, 1 showed no deterioration in the five months period of observation and in 2 progression of the disease was uninterrupted. In only 1 of this group did complete progesterone suppression occur.

The authors concluded that buserelin administered alone is helpful in the treatment of premenopausal advanced breast cancer.

Conclusions on the treatment of advanced breast cancer in the premenopausal women

By the introduction of less invasive methods of endocrinal manipulation it is possible to attain response rates in premenopausal advanced breast cancer similar to those found after surgical or irradiation-induced oophorectomy. The use of tamoxifen in this setting has produced encouraging results and the initial reports of clinical trials incorporating the use of luteinizing hormone-releasing hormone agonists are encouraging.

It is, however, important to note that at the present time such reports are preliminary and further studies are required before surgical oophorectomy is replaced as the treatment of choice.

The major advantage that these new treatments have over accepted therapy are their ease of administration and lack of toxicity, an important aspect in a disease in which only one-third of patients can be expected to respond to treatment.

References
Klijn, J.G. (1984) Long term LH/RH agonist treatment in metastatic breast cancer as a single treatment and in combination with other additive endocrine treatments. *Med. Oncol. Tumour Pharmacother., 1 No. 22,* 123–128.
Nicholson, R.I. & Maynard, P.V. (1979) Anti-tumour activity of ICI 118630, a new potent luteinizing hormone-releasing hormone agonist. *Br. J. Cancer, 39,* 268.
Pritchard, K.I., Thompson, D.B., Myers, R.E. et al (1980) Tamoxifen therapy in premenopausal patients with metastatic breast cancer. *Cancer Treatment Reports, 64,* 787–796.
Stewart, H. (1970) Oophorectomy response as an index to further endocrine ablation. In: *The Clinical Management of Advanced Breast Cancer,* ed. Joslin, C.A.F. & Gleave, E.N. pp. 12–20. Cardiff: Second Tenovus Workshop.
Wada, T., Koyama, H. & Terasawa, T. (1981) Effect of Tamoxifen in premenopausal Japanese women with advanced breast cancer. *Cancer Treatments Reports, 65 No. 7–8,* 728–729.

20 Adrenalectomy

Richard Bennett

With the availability of cortisone as replacement therapy, bilateral adrenalectomy became possible as an additional method of endocrine ablation in the management of advanced breast cancer. For many years it was used in conjunction with oophorectomy in the management of postmenopausal women, and on relapse of the disease following a previously successful oophorectomy in premenopausal women. Although a number of clinical guidelines were used to help select patients for operation, it remained difficult to predict just which women were likely to respond. The current availability of hormone receptor assays on breast cancer cells has been helpful in this regard, but the response can still not be predicted with certainty. Significant experience with the procedure has been reported by many authors.

In recent years the situation has changed further with the introduction of tamoxifen, aminoglutethimide and chemotherapeutic agents. While medical 'adrenalectomy' has its advocates the value of surgical adrenalectomy should not be forgotten.

Our own experience with a long-term follow-up of 300 patients treated by adrenalectomy showed that 38% of patients responded for at least three months and that the median duration of response was 15 months. The quality of life enjoyed by responding patients was most impressive. Virtually all responding patients enjoyed either a good or fair quality of life without any major restrictions or symptoms arising from their treatment. Another important observation was that 11% of the responders were still in remission at four years, and 10% were alive at 10 years (Fig. 20.1).

We believe that these results remain important as a yardstick, and should be carefully considered in assessing the relative merits of alternative methods of treatment, such as the use of aminoglutethimide which is discussed in the next chapter.

Problems of adrenalectomy

While surgical adrenalectomy has certainly produced many extremely satisfactory responses, the complications which are sometimes associated with operation need to be considered before making a final selection. This chapter will deal essentially with the nature and incidence of complications of adrenalectomy and also the means by which they can be avoided or minimized. As the complications of adrenalectomy are, of course, mainly related to operation, emphasis will be placed upon preoperative

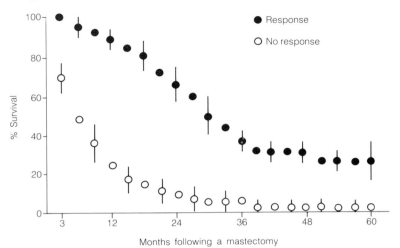

Figure 20.1
Survival of patients following bilateral adrenalectomy plus oophorectomy at the presentation of secondary disease. Graphs show survival of objective responders (38%) against non-responders.

problems and details of surgical technique. Occasional problems also relate to the adequacy of steroid replacement therapy.

Preoperative problems and potential complications

As with all surgery, operative complications can be minimized by having the patient in the best possible condition prior to surgery.

1 *Respiratory problems*

Every attention should be given to the respiratory system, particularly when this is the site of metastases. Pleural effusions should be aspirated, and if necessary intercostal tubes passed to allow complete drainage. Subsequent re-expansion of the underlying lung should be encouraged with vigorous physiotherapy. Associated pulmonary collapse and infection need to be treated vigorously with physiotherapy and the use of appropriate antibiotics. If doubt exists as to the adequacy of respiratory function, then blood gases should be estimated and the advice of a respiratory physician obtained. While pulmonary and pleural complications do not necessarily preclude adrenalectomy they certainly increase the risk, and optimal conditions should be obtained prior to surgery.

2 *Haematological problems*

A full haematological examination should be performed, and the presence of anaemia, which is not uncommon, corrected by transfusion if necessary. Thrombocytopenia and an associated bleeding tendency sometimes exist, usually in association with splenomegaly and hepatomegaly consequent to metastases. The thrombocytopenia, which is usually associated with platelet destruction within the spleen, can sometimes be corrected by planned splenectomy at the time of adrenalectomy. However, little can be done to correct the problem prior to surgery, apart from arranging for the availability of fresh blood and platelets for transfusion at the time of operation.

3 *Liver problems*
Liver dysfunction is also occasionally associated with a bleeding tendency due to a reduction in the necessary clotting factors present in the blood. If a decision is made to proceed with operation, then an attempt should be made to identify deficiencies and correct them before operation. Adequate reserves of fresh blood should be available for transfusion during the operation should this become necessary.

The presence and extent of hepatomegaly also needs to be carefully assessed. This is of special importance if an anterior approach is made to the adrenal glands, when major hepatomegaly can seriously interfere with the approach to the right adrenal gland. Under these circumstances a posterior approach may be more appropriate.

Extensive infiltration of the liver by metastases can eventually produce serious interference with liver function. This needs to be checked carefully to determine whether the liver is capable of coping with the metabolic changes and stress induced by anaesthesia and operation.

4 *Ascites*
Ascites is a bad preoperative sign. While the fluid can be released at laparotomy, and exposure is often facilitated by the lax abdominal wall, the ascites is usually associated with extensive intraperitoneal disease. The fluid may recur quickly following operation with increased risk of dehiscence of the wound. Under these circumstances it may be wise to choose a posterior approach to the adrenal glands, or, if an anterior approach is used, to add reinforcing sutures at the time of wound closure.

Operative considerations

Steroid replacement
This usually commences with the administration of hydrocortisone 100 mg intramuscularly at the time of premedication, followed by another 100 mg given intravenously during the operation. After operation, hydrocortisone is continued intravenously in doses of 100 mg six-hourly during the first day, and 50 mg six-hourly on the second day. Thereafter, the drip is usually out and replacement is continued with cortisone acetate 50 mg eight-hourly by mouth, reducing this quickly over the next two or three days to a maintenance dose of 25 mg in the morning and 12.5 mg or 25 mg in the evening, supplemented by 0.1 mg fludrocortisone acetate in the morning. Maintenance levels are usually reached after about six days, with the patient leaving hospital between the eighth and tenth day in the absence of other problems.

Approach

When the ovaries also require to be removed then the anterior transperitoneal approach has obvious advantages.

When the ovaries have already been removed then a posterior or loin approach to the adrenal glands is acceptable, and preferred by some surgeons. However, this approach certainly requires at least two incisions, and a third if it is combined with oophorectomy. When the liver is particularly enlarged, or the subcostal angle is very narrow, then the posterior approach may be easier, but my own preference is almost invariably the anterior approach. This involves one incision only, allows an adequate laparotomy as well as oophorectomy when required, and is not associated with excessive postoperative pain. In fact my experience is that the patients are more comfortable and move more freely, thus encouraging respiratory function.

The anterior approach is made through a long bilateral subcostal incision, which in effect is a transverse epigastric incision with a curve convex superiorly. While obesity certainly adds to the difficulty of exposure, I have found this less important than the presence of a very narrow subcostal angle. Fortunately, most obese patients seem to have a wide subcostal angle, and the thickened subcutaneous tissue is maximal inferiorly, so that a long incision as above will usually provide surprisingly good access. I prefer a nasogastric tube to be passed at commencement of the operation to ensure that the stomach is deflated, but I do not usually leave it in after operation.

The exposure of the right adrenal gland is more difficult than the left. The liver needs to be retracted with care, which is facilitated by the long subcostal incision. When the liver is enlarged, additional precautions are necessary. The retractor should be chosen with care and a pack placed between it and the liver to ensure that the capsule is not breached. Should this occur, then persistent oozing is likely to occur with blood running backwards into the region of the adrenal gland. Increased efforts to expose the region tend to cause further bleeding.

A pack is placed over the duodenum and the right kidney, which are both displaced downwards by the left hand of the operator. The inferior vena cava is then identified and exposed by carefully dividing the posterior parietal peritoneum vertically along the cava, and then laterally above the kidney. Dissection is concentrated on the cava which is traced carefully in a superior direction. Not infrequently, small accessory hepatic veins enter the front of the inferior vena cava from the surface of the liver. These should be identified, carefully dissected, and divided between silk ligatures. This manoeuvre increases the ease of exposure at the upper end, facilitating retraction of the liver.

Further careful dissection of the right and posterior aspects of the upper part of the cava reveals the right adrenal vein. This is usually single and passing forwards from the gland into the back of the cava. However, occasionally there are accessory veins which should also be identified. This part of the dissection needs to be done with care to avoid tearing either the adrenal vein or the inferior vena cava. Once the vein has been identified, ligatures can again be passed around it and carefully tied. Some surgeons prefer clips, but I feel much more secure with silk ties. Thereafter, the vein is divided and the gland dissected away from the cava. This is usually a simple manoeuvre but once again care should be taken with the retraction of the liver and the inferior vena cava. Sometimes small arteries are found supplying the gland, reaching it along its medial border. These are small, but if identified need to be ligated or controlled with diathermy. Without doubt the important vessel is the adrenal vein and once this has been safely divided the rest of the dissection should proceed smoothly and without undue haemorrhage.

The two problems which might therefore be encountered on the right side are exposure and haemorrhage. Exposure is greatly facilitated by the nature of the incision, the choice of retractors, division of accessory hepatic veins, and gentle traction downwards on the duodenum and left kidney. Haemorrhage must be avoided by very gentle handling of the liver and meticulous dissection of the veins joining the inferior vena cava. Should brisk haemorrhage result then immediate control with a pack is simple. The only problem is to ensure that the return of blood to the heart through the inferior vena cava is not impeded to such an extent that the blood pressure falls excessively. However, once the wound is cleared of blood and the retractor is again carefully positioned, any bleeding from the inferior vena cava should be quickly controlled with a long fine artery forcep or a curved vascular clamp. It is important that everything is in readiness for the application of the clamp before removing the pack, for repeated attempts to apply the clamp may result in further tearing of the cava. The junction of the adrenal vein with the cava, or any small tear which has developed, is then oversewn with an atraumatic suture of 3/0 silk. Clearly, prevention by good exposure and careful dissection is better than enforced suture.

Occasionally the right adrenal gland is the site of metastases, and these may be palpable at operation. Infiltration by the metastasis outside the capsule of the gland makes this adherent, sometimes to the inferior vena cava. Though it is tempting to believe that this might be more readily removed by the posterior approach, this has not been my experience. The adrenal vein always passes forwards into the back of the vena cava and when dissection is particularly difficult I have always found it better to approach the gland from in front so long as adequate exposure can be achieved.

The left adrenal gland may be approached by several methods. The first of these involves mobilization of the spleen, along with the tail and body of the pancreas, which are rotated forwards and towards the right, away from the left kidney and the left adrenal gland. While this certainly provides good exposure it is not without risk to the spleen, and splenectomy has been required in approximately one-quarter of such patients.

The gland may also be approached through the lesser sac, dividing the gastrocolic omentum anteriorly. However, this still requires mobilization of the pancreas through the lesser sac, and is, in my view, much less satisfactory than the third choice.

The approach which I prefer is through the base of the transverse mesocolon. The transverse colon is wrapped in a moist pack and held on the surface of the wound, thus tensing the transverse mesocolon. The small bowel is wrapped in a moist pack and displaced inferiorly, and the duodenojejunal flexure identified and displaced to the right side. The inferior mesenteric vein is usually identified on the left side of the fourth part of the duodenum, and avoided. Should it interfere subsequently with the dissection, it can be clamped and divided without risk. The mesocolon is divided with scissors on its inferior aspect and adjacent to the inferior mesenteric vein. This leads posteriorly into an areolar plane which can be readily opened with blunt-edged scissors or a wool dissector. Almost immediately the medial end of the left renal vein is identified. Exposure is facilitated with a narrow Dever's or a long pelvic retractor. With careful dissection it is not difficult to identify the left adrenal vein as it descends to join the left renal vein. This is usually of considerable size and should be treated with care. It is not usually difficult to clean it, following which it is divided between carefully tied ligatures. The ligature on the proximal end leads the operator to the left adrenal gland. To gain satisfactory exposure the long retractor needs to be passed through the opening in the transverse mesocolon and the pancreas, with the splenic vein on its posterior surface, should be lifted forward off the adrenal gland. Once the gland has been identified, it is dissected with long scissors, keeping close to its capsule. Almost invariably there are additional vessels along its medial border, including an artery which is larger than on the right side. This should be clamped, divided and ligated, along with any related vein. The gland is then usually dissected from the surrounding fatty and areolar tissue without difficulty, although care should be taken not to damage veins in the region of the renal hilum. When the gland has been removed haemostasis is usually secured with the aid of diathermy. It should be noted that the left adrenalectomy is performed without disturbance to the spleen and stomach, and with minimal displacement of the pancreas. No attempt is made to suture the opening in the transverse mesocolon, and under normal circumstances drainage is not necessary on either side.

If oophorectomy is necessary, the small bowel, which is wrapped in a moist pack, is simply displaced upwards while the lower margin of the wound is retracted inferiorly. Access to the pelvis and to both ovaries is usually quite adequate.

Operation is completed with minimal disturbance to the small bowel, and no traction on the small bowel mesentery. The transverse colon and greater omentum are replaced in the lower abdomen and the upper abdominal wound sutured in layers with a reinforcing suture for the linea alba. The subcutaneous tissue is approximated with catgut, and the skin with either a sub-cuticular suture or interrupted sutures according to preference. The nasogastric tube is removed at the end of the operation.

A bladder catheter is passed before operation if the ovaries are to be removed, but otherwise only if there has been some concern about the degree of blood loss or instability of blood pressure, making postoperative monitoring of urine output desirable. Whenever possible it is better to do without a catheter to avoid the possibility of a consequential urinary tract infection.

Postoperatively the intravenous line is maintained for 24–48 hours. It is rare for postoperative ileus to develop. The patient is encouraged to sit out of bed the day after operation, and also to commence taking small amounts of fluid orally if bowel sounds are present. Usually, fluids by mouth can be increased quite quickly with removal of the intravenous drip and continuation of steroid replacement by mouth. Pain relief is important to facilitate moving, breathing and coughing. However, it is surprising how little pain the transverse incisions produce and it is not difficult to ensure comfort by pethidine given either intermittently by intramuscular injection or continuously by intravenous infusion.

Postoperative problems

Every effort is made to avoid postoperative respiratory complications and deep venous thrombosis by ensuring comfort, early mobility, and vigorous breathing and coughing exercises. In patients with preoperative chest problems this is particularly important, and any preoperative treatment must be continued after operation to ensure full re-expansion of the lungs and the avoidance of sputum retention. Although these patients are theoretically at greater risk of developing thrombotic complications, it has not been my practice to administer prophylactic heparin. The transverse upper abdominal wounds usually heal quickly within the first week. I have not, on any occasion, encountered dehiscence of the wound, and incisional hernias are extremely rare. Both are clearly more likely with postoperative distension, respiratory infection, large obese patients, and the presence of preoperative ascites.

Postoperative monitoring of urine output, serum electrolytes, and haemoglobin, should be undertaken throughout the first 48 hours, and longer if necessary. Steroid replacement is provided as previously described, but increased infection or other complications occur. Before leaving hospital, the patient is instructed carefully about the need for continuing steroid replacement and for its administration by injection should persistent vomiting occur. The need for increased replacement in the presence of

Complications	Numbers	Percentages
Pulmonary complications	24	8
Wound	14	4.7
Systemic infection	2	1
Acute adrenal insufficiency	13	4.3
Chronic adrenal insufficiency	14	4.7

sepsis should also be emphasized, and the family doctor kept fully informed of progress and treatment. At postoperative visits a regular check is maintained of weight, blood pressure, urinalysis, and serum electrolytes are estimated as required. While chronic steroid depletion is not common, its onset is often insidious, and its presence should be suspected whenever the patient complains of increased weakness and loss of appetite.

In the series of 300 adrenalectomies referred to previously, the complications encountered are listed in Table 20.1. With care their incidence is not great, but their occurrence can be a major problem in a sick patient. Prevention is therefore all important. Selection of patients and thorough preoperative preparation are crucial, as are attention to operative detail and meticulous dissection. Complications remain minimal so long as rigid adherence to the above matters is maintained.

Adrenalectomy is an operation that is performed without great difficulty in experienced hands. Although there is pain over the first 24 hours, recovery is swift and usually uncomplicated (Fig. 20.2) and complications from steroid replacement are minimal. Response can be prolonged and of good quality. The exact place of adrenalectomy as a second-line endocrine therapy following tamoxifen is, as yet, undefined.

Figure 20.2
Patient on second
postoperative day.
Recovery from the
operation is rapid.

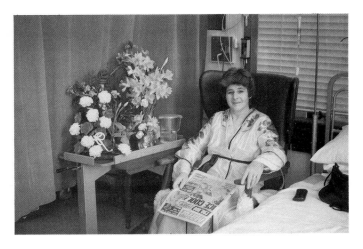

Further reading

Bennett, R.C. (1983) Long-term follow-up of surgical adrenalectomy for breast cancer. *Aust. N.Z. J. Surg.*, *53*, 415–419.

Fracchia, A.A., Randall, H.T. & Farrow, J.H. (1967) The results of adrenalectomy in advanced breast cancer in 500 consecutive patients. *Surg. Gynecol. Obstet.*, *125*, 747–756.

Horsley, J.S., Alrich, E.M., Sears, H.F. & Creighton, B.W. (1971) Adrenalectomy for metastatic mammary cancer. *Ann. Surg.*, *173*, 906–912.

Russell, I.S. & Corbet, S. (1976) The anterior approach to the adrenal gland. *Aust. N.Z. J. Surg.*, *46*, 383–387.

Silverstein, M.J., Byron, R.L., Yonemoto, R.H., Rihimaki, D.U. & Schuster, G. (1975) Bilateral adrenalectomy for advanced breast cancer: a 21 year experience. *Surgery*, *77*, 825–832.

21 The Place of Aminoglutethimide

Adrian L. Harris

Does aminoglutethimide replace adrenalectomy?
This question has already been answered in clinical practice, for surgical adrenalectomy has declined markedly in frequency as new hormonal therapy has appeared. In this chapter I will initially review and compare aminoglutethimide therapy with surgical adrenalectomy and make the case that adrenalectomy is no longer indicated in the management of breast cancer.

Of recent years tamoxifen has become the accepted first-line treatment of secondary disease in postmenopausal women in several series; aminoglutethimide has proved effective second-line therapy to tamoxifen. Response rates ranged from 15% in tamoxifen non-responders to 47% in previous tamoxifen responders. On the other hand, there is very little data and therefore no convincing evidence that adrenalectomy has a place in sequential hormone therapy after tamoxifen as first-line therapy.

Aminoglutethimide (AG), an analogue of the hypnotic glutethimide, was introduced as an anticonvulsant in 1960 (Hughes & Burley, 1970). It produced side-effects including goitre, ovarian dysfunction and adrenal insufficiency. AG was withdrawn and reintroduced as an adrenal suppressant. This has led to its use for endocrine-responsive tumours such as breast cancer, prostate cancer, endometrial cancer and adrenal overactivity of various causes.

Action of AG   AG inhibits production of steroids, particularly oestrogens. The first step in adrenal steroid biosynthesis is the conversion of cholesterol to pregnenolone. This is inhibited by AG but can be overcome by a reflex rise in adrenocorticotrophic hormone (ACTH) or exogenous ACTH. Replacement doses of hydrocortisone (20 mg twice a day) or cortisone acetate (25 mg twice a day) are given to prevent the rise in ACTH.

AG inhibits several other adrenal enzymes that contain cytochrome P450. Aldosterone levels fall by 70–80%, but substitution therapy with 0.1 mg fludrocortisone is usually only necessary in hot climates or in conditions with excessive salt loss. Enzymes on the pathway to cortisol biosynthesis may also be inhibited but cortisol deficiency in adults has not been described, even without cortisol replacement, because ACTH can overcome the blocks.

The main source of oestrogen in postmenopausal women is produced by peripheral conversion of adrenal androgens to oestrogens by aromatase AG inhibits this enzyme in vivo by 95–98%. Human breast cancers contain aromatase and may produce oestrogens locally (Miller et al, 1982). It is probable that the main site of action of AG in breast cancer is aromatase rather than adrenal inhibition. Oestrone and oestradiol levels fall by 60–80% on therapy.

Administration of AG to premenopausal women only minimally affects oestrogen production by the ovarian follicles. The effect on the menses are variable—no effect, amenorrhoea or increased frequency of bleeding.

Aminoglutethimide is well absorbed orally and is mainly excreted in the urine within 72 hours.

The standard dosage regimen has been 250 mg four times a day in divided dosage, plus hydrocortisone 20 mg twice a day.

Action of adrenalectomy

The adrenal gland does not secrete oestrogens. Adrenal androgens are the main source of oestrogens in postmenopausal women, being converted by peripheral aromatase to oestrone and oestradiol. Adrenalectomy markedly lowers androgen levels and deprives aromatase of its main substrates (testosterone and Δ4 androstenedione) and thus lowers oestradiol and oestrone levels. Other sources of androgens can help maintain oestrogen levels. The postmenopausal ovary is a significant source of androgens (Bolufer et al, 1983) and after adrenalectomy mean urinary oestrone levels are significantly higher in spontaneously menopausal patients compared with oophorectomized patients.

Comparison of aminoglutethimide with adrenalectomy in clinical practice

One of the problems in comparing AG with surgery is patient selection. Large older series of adrenalectomized patients were gradually more carefully selected as clinical indices of response were described: prolonged disease-free interval, previous response to hormone therapy, and sites of disease influenced response rate and selection. Tending to lower response rates is the observation that most patients had received other hormone therapies first. The accumulated data from eight large trials (nearly 2000 patients) showed a response rate varying from 28 to 51% (Table 21.1). In Fracchi's series of 500 patients the rate was 35.4%.

The response rates above are remarkably similar to those for aminoglutethimide in patients not selected for oestrogen receptor-positive tumours. In over 1000 patients the objective response rate is approximately 30% (range 28–53%; Table 21.1). In several of these series, patients had had extensive prior hormone or chemotherapy. With AG the length of tumour-free interval or the number of years past the menopause do not influence the response rate (Harris et al, 1983).

Patients with previous objective response to hormone therapy had a 38% response rate to AG, but only a 19% response rate if

Table 21.1
Objective response
rates to
aminoglutethimide or
adrenalectomy in
eight large series.

	% response	No. of responders
Adrenalectomy	28	455
	30	13
	35	166
	38	248
	29	27
	39	137
	41	95
	51	150
Aminoglutethimide plus hydrocortisone	28	53
	30	17
	33	30
	37	50
	37	48
	42	10
	43	19
	53	21

they had previously failed. This is similar to the results for adrenalectomy, with a 40% and 10% response rate, respectively (McDonald, 1962). The response rate in ER-positive tumours to aminoglutethimide is 56% and for adrenalectomy it is 50% (Table 21.2).

Because of the problem of patient selection, a randomized trial is the optimum way to compare treatments. The comparisons above suggest that there would be no difference and this was the result in the only randomized trial reported. The response rate to AG was 53% versus 45% for adrenalectomy (Santen et al, 1981). The median response duration in this trial was 17 months for both arms.

There is no evidence that AG is inferior to adrenalectomy in similar patients and there is the advantage that the drug therapy can be given to patients with poorer performance status, those

Table 21.2
Response to
aminoglutethimide or
adrenalectomy in
different reports in
ER-positive patients.

	No. of responders	% response
Adrenalectomy	9/17	53
	9/19	47
Aminoglutethimide plus hydrocortisone	15/22	68
	4/9	47.5
	19/38	50

with hypercalcaemia or spinal secondaries and patients with other medical problems contraindicating adrenalectomy.

Complications of the therapies

Adrenalectomy The morbidity and mortality of adrenalectomy is well recognized. In addition, lifelong replacement therapy is necessary with hydrocortisone and fludrocortisone and it is extremely difficult to mimic the normal cortisol secretion pattern. Individual patients requirements appear to vary twofold but this is often not taken into account and treatment is rarely individualized using ACTH profiles. The patient is at lifelong risk of an Addisonian crisis.

Because of the necessary surgery, many patients are excluded from therapy.

Aminoglutethimide One of the limitations on the use of AG has been its toxicity, which is similar to that of several anticonvulsants. Side-effects include nausea, vomiting, dizziness, ataxia, drowsiness and depression. Most of these side-effects are self-limiting and decrease 2–6 weeks after starting therapy. Enzyme induction may explain this. Doses are often increased gradually to avoid or reduce these initial side-effects, e.g. AG 250 mg twice daily plus hydrocortisone, is gradually increased by 250 mg every 2 weeks to 250 mg 4 times a day.

A macular-papular skin rash occurs in 25% of patients and usually resolves spontaneously after 10 days. AG does not have to be discontinued. Other side-effects include cramps, an influenza-like syndrome and, rarely, reversible neutropenia, thrombocytopenia or pancytopenia have occurred. The incidence of the latter is less than 1% and in most cases recovery occurs rapidly when administration of the drug is stopped. The reaction appears to be idiosyncratic, although most cases have had some predisposing problem with the marrow, such as infiltration or recent radiotherapy. With conventional doses of AG, 60% of patients have no side-effects, 35% have transient side-effects, and 5% cannot continue with the drug.

Adrenal function is depressed (see above) but within 36 hours of stopping AG, normal adrenal function is obtained; this includes normal stress test responses. Thyroxine (T_4) levels fall by 15% on therapy, but thyroid-stimulating hormone (TSH) rises and T_4 levels are normal 6 months after starting treatment. Myxoedema occurs in under 5% of patients (1 in 200 in our experience).

Low-dose aminoglutethimide

Because aromatase is the important site of action of AG and is much more sensitive than adrenal enzymes, low doses of AG, 125 mg twice daily with hydrocortisone, have been assessed. The incidence of rash was the same as high-dose AG, but drowsiness, nausea and ataxia were greatly reduced. In a series of 72 patients, including patients up to age 80, only 1 stopped AG. That was due to nausea and she had simultaneously started opiates. The objective response rate was the same as reported for conventional-dose AG. Low-dose AG can be considered to be the optimal way to use AG. Oestrone and oestradiol suppression is equivalent to higher doses of AG.

Conclusions

There is no clinical or biochemical criterion that shows adrenalectomy to be superior to AG. Because AG, particularly low-dose AG, is well tolerated, rapidly reversible and can be administered to any patient, in the opinion of this author, it clearly should replace adrenalectomy. To subject 50% of patients having adrenalectomy to unnecessary surgery and lifelong replacement therapy, and possibly malaise due to inadequate cortisol replacement, is, in my view, unnecessary. A trial of endocrine therapy with low-dose AG and hydrocortisone can be recommended as second-line treatment after tamoxifen or as first-line treatment for multiple bone secondaries.

Further reading

Bolufer, P., Antonio, P., Carcia, R. et al (1983) Role of the ovary in the regulation of sex hormone binding globulin and its contribution to peripheral levels of androstenedione. *Exp. Clin. Endocrinol.*, *82*, 29.

Cantwell, B.M.J., Sainsbury, J.R.C., Harris, A.L. et al (1984) Low dose aminoglutethimide. Phase II study in advanced postmenopausal breast cancer. *Br. J. Cancer*, *50*, 252.

Fracchi, A.A., Farrow, J.H., Miller, T.R. et al (1971) Hypophysectomy as compared with adrenalectomy in the treatment of advanced carcinoma of the breast. *Surg. Gynecol. Obstet.*, *133*, 241.

Grodin, J.M., Siiteri, P.K. & MacDonald, P.C. (1973) Source of estrogen production in postmenopausal women. *J. Clin. Endocrinol. Metab.*, *36*, 207.

Harris, A.L., Powles, T.J., Smith, I.E. et al (1983) Aminoglutethimide for the treatment of advanced postmenopausal breast cancer. *Eur. J. Cancer Clin. Oncol.*, *19*, 11.

Hughes, S.W.M. & Burley, D.M. (1970) Aminoglutethimide. A 'side-effect' turned to therapeutic advantage. *Postgrad. Med. J.*, *46*, 409.

McDonald, I. (1962) Endocrine ablation in disseminated mammary carcinoma. *Surg. Gyn. Obstet.*, *115*, 215.

Miller, W.R., Hawkins, R.A. & Forrest, A.P.M. (1982) Significance of aromatase activity in human breast cancer. *Cancer Res.*, *42 (Suppl.)*, 3365S.

Santen, R.J., Worgul, T.J., Samojlik, E. et al (1981) A randomized trial comparing surgical adrenalectomy with aminoglutethimide plus hydrocortisone in women with advanced breast cancer. *N. Engl. J. Med.*, *305*, 545.

22 Chemotherapy

Richard Blake

Although chemotherapy has been used in the treatment of advanced breast cancer for more than 20 years, little comparative data exists of differing drug regimens or of the possible benefit to patients in terms of survival. Most reports have been concerned about response rates with little information about actuarial survival data. Powles et al (1980) maintained that over the previous ten-year period there had been no improvement in survival of patients from the appearance of their first metastasis and reported that in some patients chemotherapy had shortened life.

The evaluation and comparison of differing chemotherapy regimens is possible in centres which have an interest in the management of breast cancer. For the clinician in a district general hospital who may not be participating in clinical trials, patients receiving chemotherapy require careful supervision and treatment should be carried out preferably by clinicians experienced in the use of these drugs.

This chapter will consider the assessment of patients receiving chemotherapy and report the Nottingham experience of systemic chemotherapy in patients with advanced breast cancer.

Assessment

It is of upmost importance that women receiving chemotherapy should be assessed prior to the start and during treatment. Patients should be evaluated as to response, duration of remission and survival. Side-effects of therapy should be recorded and a judgement made of the patient's quality of life.

Standard criteria for assessment of response have been described by the British Breast Group and the International Union against Cancer (UICC). Objective methods used to assess disease are clinical measurements, photography of lesions, laboratory investigations and the selective use of radiology, ultrasound and radioisotope scanning. The UICC categories of response are:

1 Complete response; disappearance of all known disease with sclerosis of lytic bone metastases.
2 Partial response; at least 50% reduction in measurable lesions with no new lesions appearing.
3 Static; lesions unchanged.
4 Progressive disease; progression and/or appearance of new lesions.

Many factors may affect a patient's ability to tolerate treatment and a careful monitoring of the side-effects is necessary prior to each course of cytotoxic therapy. Side-effects are better tolerated if there is evidence of tumour response, but if there is progressive disease treatment should either be stopped or an alternative chemotherapy regimen considered. It behoves the clinician to avoid subjecting patients to the side-effects of cytotoxic treatment which is having no tumouricidal effect.

The quality of life during chemotherapy can be assessed subjectively or an attempt at objective measurement can be made using the Karnofsky system or a scoring system such as the Linear Analogue Self Assessment where patients mark a line at intervals according to how they rated various symptoms.

Drugs

Chemotherapeutic agents may be used singly or in combination, the two most effective single agents appearing to be cyclophosphamide and doxorubicin with response rates of 30–50%. 5-Fluorouracil, methotrexate, vincristine, phenylalanine mustard can be used as single agents, but in recent years, as with other solid tumours, many regimens have been described using these drugs in various combinations. Most drug combinations use cyclophosphamide and/or doxorubicin with the addition of other agents. Recently introduced agents which need evaluation in the treatment of breast cancer are ifosfamide, an analogue of cyclophosphamide, mitozantrone and epiadriamycin.

Toxicity of these drugs which often require reduction or cessation of treatment causes nausea, vomiting, alopecia and marrow suppression. Other less common side-effects are oral ulceration, chemical cystitis and a peripheral neuropathy. Combination regimens are designed using drugs with different modes of action and toxicity in the hope of an increased tumouricidal effect without increasing toxicity. The combination of cyclophosphamide, methotrexate, 5-Fluorouracil, vincristine and prednisolone (CMFVP) comprise the original 'Cooper' regimen and was reported to produce a response rate of over 90%. Despite this initial favourable response later reports using a modified regimen have shown a response of about 60–70% sustained for three months and falling to about 50% at six months (Edelstyn et al, 1979).

At the City Hospital in Nottingham we have treated a consecutive number of women with advanced breast cancer using differing drug regimens over a 12-year period. We initially used a modified 'Cooper' regimen (Wilson et al, 1979), but were encouraged by a report by Priestman and Salaman (1978) on the use of oral melphalan and methotrexate which appears to have little toxicity. We subsequently used the single agent, cyclophosphamide, in high dosage.

Nottingham experience

A consecutive series of 187 patients with advanced breast cancer were referred for chemotherapy. These patients included those who had previously undergone mastectomy and those who presented with a primary inoperable breast cancer.

All patients referred for chemotherapy had had prior endocrine treatment apart from a small group of 20 women from earlier in the series who had been defined as a Dire Prognostic Group (DPG) unlikely to respond to endocrine therapy. This DPG group had either liver metastases, intraperitoneal metastases, CNS metastases or metastases in three separate tissues; such patients had been shown by Cutler et al (1969) to have a short life expectancy and it was thought reasonable to omit endocrine therapy. This policy was later abandoned and all patients referred thereafter had received prior endocrine therapy and had either failed to respond or had shown a response and then relapsed from control. All patients were seen at a chemotherapy clinic for their assessment, treatment and follow-up.

The chemotherapy regimens used are shown in Table 22.1. All patients were given treatment on an out-patient basis requiring one to two visits each month, except those patients receiving high-dose cyclophosphamide who were admitted to hospital for two to three days. Treatment was given at the dosages shown, unless the white blood cell count (WBC) had fallen to less than 3.0×10^9/litre and/or their platelet count had fallen to less than 90×10^9/litre, when treatment was withheld for a period of two to three weeks. Treatment was resumed after this period if blood counts were satisfactory. If subsequent haematological toxicity occurred, then further dosage was reduced by 25%. Gastrointestinal side-effects were managed by antiemetics and antidiarrhoeal agents and wigs were prescribed if necessary. If intolerable side-effects occurred then treatment was stopped.

Table 22.1
Chemotherapy regimens used in Nottingham.

1. CMFVP regimen
Cyclophosphamide: 2.5 mg/kg/day orally (days 1–14)
Methotrexate: 0.3 mg/kg
5-Fluorouracil: 15 mg/kg   intravenously (days 1 and 8)
Vincristine: 0.015 mg/kg
Prednisolone: 5 mg t.d.s. orally, continuously
Cycle repeated on day 29 to a total of 6 cycles

2. Melphalan and methotrexate
melphalan: 15 mg (day 1)
Methotrexate: 10 mg (daily for 5 days)
Cycle repeated every 6 weeks to a total of 6 cycles

3. Cyclophosphamide regimen
50 mg/kg 6 doses intravenously at 3-weekly intervals

Table 22.2
Nottingham Series: Response according to age and tumour state.

	No.	Responders
Age (years)		
< 40	14	6 (42.9%)
40–60	81	25 (30.9%)
> 60	51	10 (19.6%)
(Combining patients < 60 years)		$\chi^2 = 2.78$, df = 2, NS
Menopausal state		
Premenopausal	46	19 (41.3%)
Postmenopausal	100	22 (22.0%)
		$\chi^2 = 5.81$, $P < 0.025$
Tumour grade		
I & II	32	10 (31.3%)
III	54	20 (37.0%)
(Unknown in 60 cases)		$\chi^2 = 0.23$, NS
*Oestrogen receptors****		
< 5	36	12 (33.3%)
> 5	32	8 (25.0%)
(Unknown in 78 cases)		$\chi^2 = 0.57$, NS
Primary operable and inoperable disease		
Operable	114	35 (30.7%)
Inoperable	32	6 (18.8%)
(Unknown in 78 cases)		$\chi^2 = 1.77$, NS

** fmol/mg cytosol protein.

Table 22.3
Nottingham Series: Response according to regimen, referral group and DFI.

	No.	Responders
Drug regimen		
CMFVP	82	28 (34.1%)
M & M	35	2 (5.7%)
Cyclo.	29	11 (37.9%)
(CMFVP versus M & M)		$\chi^2 = 10.4$, df = 1, $P < 0.005$
(Cyclophosphamide versus M & M)		$\chi^2 = 10.2$, df = 1, $P < 0.005$
Referral group		
Dire Prognostic Group	20	7 (35.0%)
Failed endocrine	105	27 (25.7%)
Relapsed endocrine	21	7 (33.3%)
		$\chi^2 = 1.05$, df = 2, NS
Disease-free interval (DFI)		
0–12 (months)	41	15 (36.6%)
13–24	38	11 (28.9%)
25–36	10	3 (30.0%)
> 36	20	5 (25.0%)
(Combining patients with DFI > 24 months)		$\chi^2 = 0.93$, df = 2, NS

Table 22.4
Nottingham Series:
Response according
site of disease and no.
of sites.

	No.	Responders
Locoregional	63	18 (28.6%)
Bone	56	11 (19.6%)
Distal nodes	34	14 (41.2%)
Liver	23	6 (26.1%)
Solid lung	22	7 (31.8%)
Pleura	17	5 (21.4%)
Opposite breast	15	4 (26.7%)
Distal skin	9	3 (33.3%)
Marrow	7	2 (28.6%)
Lung—lymphangitis	6	0
Peritoneal	5	0
CNS	5	3
Pericardium	2	1
Patients with 1 site	67	18 (26.9%)
Patients with 2 sites	47	14 (29.8%)
Patients with 3 sites	27	8 (29.6%)
Patients with 4 sites	4	1 (25.0%)
Patients with 6 sites	1	0

264 tissues involved in 146 patients.

Life-table analyses and log-rank tests have been used to compare the survival rates between responding and non-responding patients. Toxicity of treatment and patterns of recurrent disease have been recorded. A chi-square test has been used for comparison of proportions.

Of 187 women who were started on chemotherapy, 41 patients died within two months of the start of treatment and were thus excluded from the analysis; it was considered that their disease was too far advanced on commencing treatment and that too few treatments had been given for the therapy to have a chance of effect. One hundred and forty-six patients have thus been analysed and 41 patients had either a complete or a partial response according to UICC criteria (an overall response of 28.1%). The non-responders either had static or progressive disease.

There was no difference in the response rates of those patients receiving either CMFVP or high-dose cyclophosphamide, but both these two regimens had significantly better response rates than the regimen of melphalan and methotrexate (Table 22.3). Analysis of various factors between responding and non-responding patients shows no clear group of women who are likely to respond to treatment (Tables 22.2, 22.3, 22.4). There is a trend for younger women to have a greater chance of response to chemotherapy and there is a significant difference in response favouring premenopausal women (Table 22.2). However, the site of

	CMFVP group (n = 82)	*M & M group* (n = 35)	*Cyclo group* (n = 29)
Mild alopecia	15 (18%)	4 (11%)	—
Severe alopecia (wig)	28 (34%)	2 (6%)	20 (69%)
Nausea and vomiting	25 (30%)	6 (17%)	22 (76%)
Diarrhoea	—	—	2 (7%)
Marrow suppression	13 (16%)	6 (17%)	—
Cystitis	5 (6%)	—	4 (14%)
Oral ulceration	3 (4%)	3 (9%)	
Peripheral neuropathy	10 (12%)	—	—
Severe infection	1 herpes 1 pneumonia	1 herpes 1 moniliasis	2 chest 2 septicaemia

Table 22.5
Nottingham Series:
Side-effects of
chemotherapy.

disease, the number of sites involved by disease, the tumour grade, the oestrogen receptor status of the primary tumour, and a previous response to endocrine treatment, have no predictive value as to the likelihood of a response to chemotherapy.

Table 22.5 shows a comparison of toxicity of the three regimens. The main side-effects of treatment were alopecia, nausea and vomiting and were more severe in the cyclophosphamide regimen. Melphalan and methotrexate had less side-effects but this regimen had a disappointing low response rate.

Figure 22.1 shows the life-table comparison of the survival rates of responding and non-responding patients, showing survival from the start of chemotherapy. The difference between the median survival between the two groups is 11 months.

Figure 22.1
Life-table comparison
of survival from start
of chemotherapy of
responders versus
non-responders.
Median survival 20
months (responders)
and 9 months (non-
responders)
($\chi^2 = 18.49$;
$P < 0.0005$).

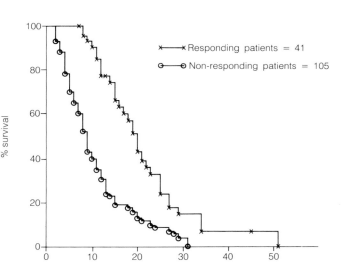

Time from commencement of cytotoxic therapy (months)

Prevention of complications

Nausea and vomiting
A number of antiemetic agents have been used for the nausea induced by cytotoxic drugs. One of the problems in the evaluation of these is that nausea and vomiting may have a variety of origins, e.g. psychological vomiting prior to administration of the chemotherapeutic drugs. Different origins (Borison and Wang, 1953) may require different treatments. Cunningham et al (1985) suggest chlorpromazine 25 mg four-hourly for 12 hours; Neidhart et al (1981) noted haloperidol as effective overall, but that their patients receiving doxorubicin preferred benzquinamide.

Hair loss
In patients receiving doxorubicin this side-effect may be lessened or prevented by effective scalp cooling (Anderson et al, 1981).

Cystitis
Patients receiving cyclophosphamide or ifosfamide are given Uromitexan (mesna) by intravenous injection. This substance protects the bladder mucosa from inflammation caused by acriline, a metabolite of oxazaphosphorines, by detoxifying acriline in the urinary tract.

Conclusions
These results show that only a small proportion of women with advanced breast cancer will benefit from chemotherapy. It is arguable whether a short period of remission of 11 months is worth while if at the same time the side-effects of treatment debilitate the patient and impair the quality of life. This said, there are certain patients in whom chemotherapy should be given for symptom relief: first among these are probably women with dyspnoea caused by pulmonary infiltration of the tumour.

Unfortunately, the majority of patients will not respond to therapy and will suffer the side-effects of treatment. It is in this group that careful assessment is important with a view to stopping treatment or considering a second-line regimen, but in our experience once a patient has relapsed she is unlikely to respond to a second-line regimen.

After our initial experience of using the combination regimen CMFVP, we have been unable to achieve any improved response using cyclophosphamide in high dosage and at the cost of increased toxicity. At present we are evaluating low-dose regimens and slow-injection administration.

Unfortunately at present there is no means of determining by clinical course, tumour characteristics, site of disease, or by biochemical indices which tumours are likely to respond to chemotherapy. The justification of using chemotherapy is that a group of women could be defined as being likely to respond to therapy. This is only likely to be achieved in centres treating large numbers of women. The future of successful cytotoxic therapy lies in the discovery of more effective and less toxic drugs.

Future advances in breast cancer chemotherapy may come from:

1 The identification of factors to predict which individual tumours are biologically capable of responding to chemotherapeutic agents.
2 The introduction of agents with greater action against breast cancer.
3 The finding of specific circulating markers of breast cancer mass in order that the chemotherapeutic effect may be judged, and agent and dosage 'titrated' against the markers.
4 A re-evaluation of the case of single-dose agents in sequence in comparison with combination regimens.

We are at present evaluating low-dose, single agents, given in sequential regimens. The hypothesis is that the reaction to cytotoxic agents is more dependent on the biology of the tumour than upon the systemic dose administered. If a tumour is sensitive, then it may be sensitive to quite a low dose and gain comparatively little from a greatly increased dose. We do not yet have fully evaluable results regarding response rates but we can say that responses have been seen. Initially ifosfamide is used, 2.5 g/m^2 given at three-weekly intervals for three doses. If the tumour has responded or remains static, then the treatment is continued until progression. If there is tumour progression then we change to another non-toxic agent, Novantrone (mitazantrone 14 mg/m^2) given for three months; the final single agent in the sequence is low-dose doxorubicin (50 mg/m^2).

Toxicity of mitazantrone has been especially low. Mitazantrone and doxorubicin are given in out-patients. To protect the bladder mesna is added to ifosfamide: this is given at 2–4 g/m^2 intravenously. The patient is therefore admitted and since this regimen gives nausea and vomiting for around 12 hours, the patient usually stays for one night. Recently, disposable slow-injection syringes have become available and we are now starting to give this regimen at the home.

Side-effects in terms of nausea and vomiting are certainly lessened using slow-injection syringes. This may lead to a reinvestigation of higher-dose regimens given over several days.

Controversies and Future Developments

- Less toxic regimens: design and evaluation.
- Prediction of response.
- Evaluation of benefit against side-effects: with the exception of certain cases (e.g., carcinomatous lymphangitis of the lung) is chemotherapy justified at all in advanced breast cancer?

References

Anderson, J.E., Hunt, J.M. & Smith, I.E. (1981) Prevention of doxorubi-
cin-induced alopecia by scalp cooling in patients with advanced breast
cancer. *Br. Med. J.*, *282*, 423–424.

Borison, H. & Wang, S.C. (1953) Physiology and pharmacology of
vomiting. *Pharmacol. Rev.*, *5*, 193–227.

British Breast Group (1974) Assessment of response to treatment in
advanced breast cancer. *Lancet, ii*, 38–39.

Cooper, R.S. (1969) Combination chemotherapy in hormone-resistant
breast cancer. *Proc. Am. Ass. Cancer Res.*, *10*, 15.

Cunningham, D., Sonkop, M., Gilchrist, N.L. et al. (1985) Randomized
trial of intravenous high dose metaclopramide and intramuscular
chlorpromazine in controlled nausea and vomiting induced by cytotoxic drugs. *Br. Med. J.*, *290*, 604–605.

Cutler, S.J., Black, M.M., Mork, T., Harvei, S. & Freeman, C. (1969)
Further observations on prognostic factors in cancer of the female
breast. *Cancer*, *24*, 653–667.

Edelstyn, G.A., Bates, T.D., Brinkley, D. et al (1979) Comparison of 5-day
and 2-day cyclical combination chemotherapy in advanced breast
cancer. *Clin. Oncol.*, *5*, 163–167.

Hayward, J.L., Rubens, R.D., Carbone, P.P. et al (1977) Assessment of
response to therapy in advanced breast cancer. *Br. J. Cancer*, *35*, 292–
298.

Karnofsky, D.A. & Burchenal, J.H. (1948) Clinical evaluation of
chemotherapeutic agents in cancer. In: *Evaluation of Chemotherapeutic Agents*, ed. MacLeod, C.M. p. 191. London: Columbia University
Press.

Neidhart, I.A., Gragen, M., Young, D. & Wilson, H.E. (1981) Specific
antiemetics for specific cancer chemotherapeutic agents. *Cancer*, *47*,
1439–1443.

Powles, T.J., Coombes, R.C., Smith, I.E. et al (1980) Failure of chemotherapy to prolong survival in a group of patients with metastatic
breast cancer. *Lancet, i*, 580–582.

Priestman, T.G. & Salaman, P.F. (1978) Melphalan and methotrexate in
advanced breast cancer. *Cancer Treatment Reports, 62, No. 12*, 2111–
2112.

Wilson, R.G., Blamey, R.W., Benton, F.M., Hardcastle, J.D. & Haybittle,
J.L. (1979) Combination chemotherapy in breast cancer: response rate
and attempts to predict response. *Clin. Oncol.*, *5*, 169–174.

23 The Management of Pain in Secondary Breast Cancer

Susan Mann

Pain is a significant component of secondary breast cancer for most patients at some stage of their illness. Eighty-five to 100% of patients with secondary breast cancer will at some time have pain that will limit their normal activity. Treatable pain is underdiagnosed in patients with secondary breast cancer. Referral of patients to a pain specialist for treatment occurs only when pain is severe, unless active assessment of pain is part of the routine assessment of these patients. Five per cent of patients from our secondary breast cancer out-patients were treated in the pain-relief clinic the year prior to a pain specialist joining the breast cancer team. During the next year, 39.4% of patients in the clinic were successfully treated for significant pain.

Assessment
Cancer patients recognize pain as part of their disease and rarely overstate its severity. An objective measurement of pain, e.g. a visual analogue scale for pain or a McGill Pain Questionnaire, is useful in conjunction with a thorough history of activity, sleep patterns, and any alteration of normal activity due to pain. Continuing assessment is necessary if maximum pain control is to be maintained.

Classification of pain
Pain may be either acute or chronic. Pain associated with cancer is associated with pathophysiological events found in chronic and recurrent pain states. Acute pain is primarily due to surgical intervention, bony collapse or rapid expansion of tumour mass. Chronic cancer pain is usually due to nociceptors in deep somatic and visceral tissue being continuously stimulated by activation of C fibres which give rise to long-term pain. Changes in the A (delta) nerve fibres include a decreased threshold giving rise to an increasing pain sensation with decreasing stimulation. This is partly due to increased prostaglandin which potentiates the effects of all noxious agents at the nociceptor by a factor of 20–50 times the normal. Decreased endorphin levels in the central nervous system are consistently found in chronic pain states. Therefore the patient with uncontrolled chronic pain is more

susceptible to acute pain. Acute pain is therefore often superimposed on a background of chronic pain. As with all chronic pain states, 'cancer pain' may continue as a 'causalgia' type pain after removal of the noxious stimuli.

Distribution of pain
The distribution of the pain is important in ascertaining the cause and best form of treatment. Discrete, local pain is often due to local soft-tissue metastases or single bony recurrences. Discrete nerve lesions can give small areas of intense pain whether they are due to involvement of peripheral nerves, nerve plexuses, nerve roots; often secondary to compression due to soft tissue or bony metastases. Referred pain at some distance from the involved nerve root is not unusual.

Regional pain may be due to bony metastases, especially of the pelvis and spine, or from tumour involvement of the central nervous system. Rapidly expanding metastases in the abdomen or chest may cause widespread visceral pain. Regional pain usually indicates a more central nervous involvement, e.g. spinal cord compression secondary to vertebral collapse, and/or more extensive tissue damage.

Generalized pain is often associated with rapidly progressing multiple metastases, although the degree of pain does not always correlate well with the speed of progression of disease. Widespread disease may lower the pain threshold as in other chronic pain states so that pain continues in spite of good tumour response to therapy.

Treatment (Figure 23.1)
Open discussion about pain and treatment goals does much to alleviate the anxiety associated with pain and the misconceptions many patients have about pain therapy. The psychological impact of 'cancer pain' cannot be overemphasized. Patient understanding, acceptance, and participation in pain control allows lower drug dosages and less aggressive management than would otherwise be possible.

Drugs   Most patients can achieve improvement, if not complete resolution of pain, with drug therapy. Adjustments to the drug regimen are required, but adequate control can be maintained with minimal side-effects by treating any increases in pain promptly and adequately. Disease progression may dictate other forms of pain therapy, but a background maintenance analgesia is often essential to maintain reasonable activity.

Non-steroidal anti-inflammatory drugs (NSAID) are effective both in mild pain and for background analgesia in moderate and several pain. In addition to some central action, one of their main contributions is a decrease in prostaglandin synthesis. This effectively raises the threshold for nociceptor stimulation. NSAID are particularly effective in patients with bone metas-

Figure 23.1
Diagram illustrating
methods of pain
control in breast
cancer.

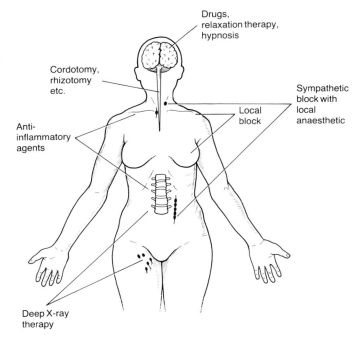

Drugs,
relaxation therapy,
hypnosis

Cordotomy,
rhizotomy
etc.

Sympathetic
block with
local
anaesthetic

Local
block

Anti-
inflammatory
agents

Deep X-ray
therapy

tases. As with all drugs, the best compound must be found for
each patient, but ibuprofen, often initially in high doses, and
indomethacin suppositories have proven effective, as has soluble
aspirin. Other analgesics, such as nefopam, are useful although
they act more centrally.

Other adjuvants include antidepressants, anticonvulsants,
and neurolepts. Small doses of antidepressants (e.g. 25 mg
amitriptyline t.d.s., or 50–75 mg *nocte*) not only aid in the
psychological adjustment needed by patients with cancer pain,
but alter pain perception. Neurolept agents (such as chlorpromazine or related compounds) in relatively small, minimally-
sedating, doses raise the pain threshold by direct opiate-agonis-
tic activity and act synergistically with antidepressants to
inhibit pain via the noradrenergic and seratonergic pathways.
Anticonvulsants, such as sodium valproate or carbamazepine,
may be useful when discrete nerve irritation can be demonstrated
(such as brachial plexus pain), and when pain persists after the
noxious stimulus has ceased, as with resolution of tumour with
therapy.

Opiate drugs constitute a significant part of the pain regimen
for most patients at some time in their treatment. As part of an
individualized programme for pain control, their side-effects can
be kept at a minimum and few problems should occur with even
long-term usage. Emphasis must be placed on pain control, rather
than 'as needed' analgesia, and in this context long-acting

opiates, which can be given orally b.d., allow many patients to lead a reasonably active life with good pain control and without frequent medication (3–4-hourly).

Temporary peripheral and regional nerve blocks

Afferent blockade central to the origin of the painful stimulus is effective for both chronic and acute pain. Appropriate local-anaesthetic block can provide adequate relief while drug therapy is adjusted or commenced, can act as a useful adjunct in controlling acute exacerbations of pain, and can aid in breaking the chronic pain cycle.

Discrete peripheral nerve lesions in secondary breast cancer are uncommon but when present respond well to anaesthetic block. Pain due to vertebral secondaries often responds well to local block. Many nerve blocks can safely be carried out on an out-patient basis, with suitable facilities for treatment of side-effects, and with the patient remaining in clinic for a suitable observation period. The most frequently used blocks include intercostal nerve blocks, interscaline blocks, suprascapular blocks, and facetal nerve blocks.

The use of intermittent or continuous epidural blockade necessitates the patient being an in-patient for a short period. Subcutaneous tunnelling of the epidural cannula can be done under local anaesthesia, and the patient can return home with the epidural in situ. Properly selected patients can do well with home administration of the analgesic agent through the cannula. Alternatively, epidural electrodes, which stimulate the pain-inhibiting pathways, can be implanted under X-ray control and give good out-patient pain control in otherwise intractable cases.

Sympathetic blockage with local anaesthetic can give long periods of relief in appropriate patients. Stellate ganglion block can be performed in the out-patient clinic, whereas lumbar synpathectomy should be performed under X-ray control. These patients, however, should not need to be admitted unless complications or side-effects of the block occur.

Destructive lesions

Pain not responsive to non-invasive pain therapy or tumour therapy may be treated with destructive nerve lesions to allow better pain control with less alteration of consciousness. Although destructive lesions by definition are invasive and can cause severe side-effects, they should not be reserved for the terminal patient. An example of a type of case suited to this is the patient with severe arm pain from brachial plexus involvement with carcinoma. The incidence of side-effects varies with the lesion and the benefit of the pain relief to the patient with intractable pain far outweighs the side-effects. Percutaneous lesions created with a radiofrequency generator range from peripheral (as intercostal) lesions and posterior rhizolysis to carotomy. The A delta and C fibres are selectively destroyed with this method and therefore preserve normal sensory and motor function. Blocks using absolute alcohol or phenol are less selective in their nerve destruction and may cause considerable side-effects; their use is now limited with the availability of the more selective methods of lesion generation. Neurosurgical techniques of nerve disruption may still be useful although again their lack of selectivity carries greater morbidity than with radiofrequency generated lesions. Pituitary ablation remains a useful form of therapy in selected patients but is rarely used since the techniques of ablation by transsphenoidal injection of absolute alcohol or radiofrequency lesion generation are less invasive and have less perioperative morbidity associated with them.

Radiotherapy   Deep X-ray therapy is of immense use, especially with bone metastases. Its limitations lie in the limitations imposed by safe dosage and the occasional pain induced by the radiotherapy. By co-ordinating other methods of pain relief with use of radiotherapy maximum benefit of radiotherapy can be produced.

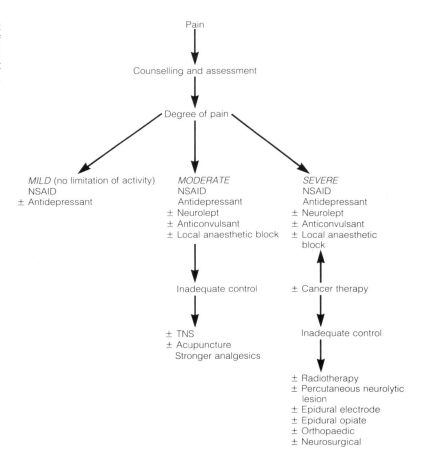

Figure 23.2
Flow diagram of approach to control of pain in breast cancer.

Non-invasive adjuncts   Transcutaneous electrical nerve stimulation, acupuncture, and hypnosis allow flexibility in the pain therapy programme for each patient. Drug dosages and the need for invasive treatment may be decreased by their utilization. The overall quality of pain control is improved by the use of simple relaxation techniques. Small alterations in pain levels can often be controlled without changes in drug regimen. The immense psychological benefit of the self-confidence felt by the patients when they can participate in controlling the pain is no small advantage in the overall treatment of the patient.

Conclusions

Any extension of life expectancy without the maintenance of quality of life is of little benefit to the patient with secondary breast cancer. At some stage of their disease they are likely to have pain that interferes with their normal activity. With greater understanding of pain mechanisms the choices for treatment with fewer side-effects have increased greatly. To achieve the best quality of life for each patient requires active assessment of pain and a multidisciplinary approach (Fig. 23.2) to the patients with the pain being seen as part of the overall problem. Most pain, if not all, can be alleviated by a humanitarian approach to the application of modern techniques for pain control. Early recognition and alleviation of pain are essential if the quality of life is to be maintained and inclusion of a pain specialist in the breast cancer team affords the greatest chance of control of pain.

Controversies and Future Developments   • The ready availability of a pain consultant in clinics for secondary breast cancer (a future reason for specialist breast clinics).

Further reading

Bonica, U. (1982) Management of cancer pain. *Acta Anaes. Scand. Suppl., 74*, 75–82.

Doyle, D. (1982) Nerve blocks in advanced cancer. *Practice of Medicine, 226*, 539–544.

Puig, M.M., Laorden, M.L., Miralles, F.S. & Olaso, M.J. (1982) Endorphin levels in cerebrospinal fluid of patients with postoperative and chronic pain. *Anaesthesiology, 57(1)*, 1–4.

Saunders, C. (1963) The treatment of intractable pain in terminal cancer. *Proc. Royal Soc. Med., 56*, 195–197.

Siegfried, J. & Krayenbuhl, H. (1982) Clinical experience in the treatment of intractable pain. In: *Pain*, ed. Janzen, R., Krudel, W.D., Herz, A. & Steichele, C. pp. 216–218. Stuttgart: Thieme.

Sindou, M., Fischer, G. & Mansug, L. (1976) Posterior spinal rhizatomy and selective rhizodiotomy. *Prog. Neurol. Surg., 7*, 201–250.

Spiegel, D. & Bloom, J. (1983) Pain in metastatic breast cancer. *Cancer, 52*, 341–345.

24 Fracture

Charles Galasko

Skeletal metastases occur frequently in patients with mammary carcinoma and may present in several ways.

- Pain (discussed in Chapter 23).
- Hypercalcaemia (discussed in Chapter 29).
- Impending fracture.
- Pathological fracture.
- Compression of the cord or cauda equina (discussed in Chapter 25).
- Spinal instability

Pathological fractures do not only affect the appendicular skeleton; spinal instability may result from bone destruction secondary to metastatic disease and is the equivalent of a pathological fracture in the appendicular skeleton.

Impending fractures

Large lytic metastases usually present with pain and the lesion is evident on X-ray. Skeletal metastases develop in the medulla and are not seen on X-ray until at least 50% of bone, in the beam axis of the X-ray, has been destroyed (Edelstyn et al, 1967). However, by the time a large lytic metastasis has developed, there is considerable bone destruction and the cortex has been involved. The mechanism of pain in these large lytic lesions is not fully understood but may be associated with infractions of the surrounding bone. The risk of fracture is high. Fidler (1973) found that if more than 50% of the cortex of a long bone was involved, there was a 50% risk of spontaneous fracture. Radiotherapy relieves pain, but temporarily weakens the bone, probably due to the associated transient osteoporosis and, as a result, may increase the risk of pathological fracture. Fourteen per cent of the pathological fractures in our series occurred through large lytic metastases that had been treated by irradiation.

Primary internal stabilization of the weakened bone has certain advantages. It is easier to fix the bone while it is still intact, and the rehabilitation and convalescence are much shorter and easier. It is the author's view that internal stabilization should be the primary treatment, followed by irradiation. The type of internal stabilization will depend on the site of the lesion. Where feasible, closed intramedullary nailing is preferred (Fig. 24.1) and, if indicated, a biopsy can be taken through a separate incision. However, intramedullary nailing may not be

Figure 24.1
Large lytic metastasis, right femur. Treated by closed intramedullary Küntscher nailing followed by radiotherapy.

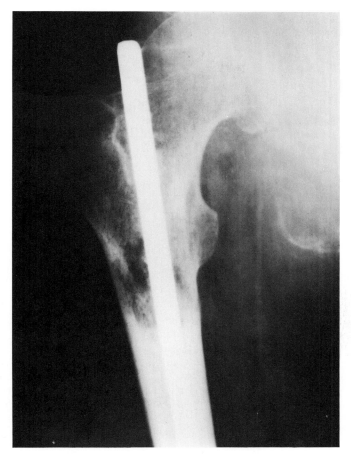

adequate at the ends of the long bones. With the exception of the femoral neck and humeral neck, the type of fixation is similar to that used for pathological fractures (see below). Large lytic metastases at these sites should be treated by internal stabilization, whereas pathological fractures of the femoral neck, and frequently of the humeral neck, are best treated by prosthetic replacement (see below).

It is essential that the internal stabilization of the lesion provides sufficient strength to allow unsupported use of the limb, including weight-bearing in the lower limb. If the implant is not likely to provide this, the stabilization should be supplemented with methylmethacrylate. The tumour is removed, the cavity filled with methylmethacrylate, while still soft, and the implant fixed across the methylmethacrylate as well as the normal bone above and below the lesion.

Irradiation is an essential part of the treatment to inhibit further tumour growth, since such growth will result in progres-

Figure 24.2
Patient with
disseminated
mammary carcinoma.
(a) Subtrochanteric
femoral fracture. (b)
Stabilized with a
blade plate. (c)
Pathological fracture
below the plate nine
months later. Had this
lesion been
demonstrated at the
time of the initial
fracture, a Zickel nail
would have been
indicated.

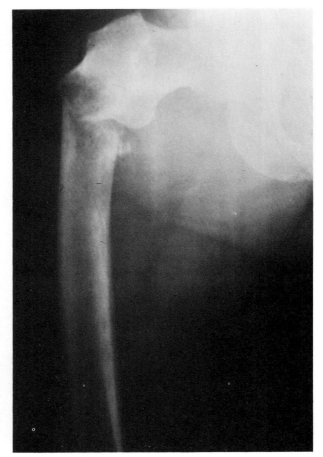

a

sive bone destruction and resultant loosening of the stabilization
with increased risk of fracture.

Internal fixation carries the theoretical risk of disseminating
tumour cells both locally and into the circulation. However, this
has never been proven, providing the lesion is irradiated.
Campbell (1967) found no radiographic or histological evidence
of spread along the tract of intramedullary rods, and many other
authors have reported no evidence of local dissemination.
Furthermore, there is no evidence that the combined effect of
surgical intervention and general anaesthesia has affected the
overall prognosis in these patients.

It also is important that, prior to treatment, scintigrams and X-
rays are obtained of the entire length of the affected bone so that
any other metastases, which may subsequently develop into a
pathological fracture, can be stabilized (Fig. 24.2) and are
included in the radiotherapy field. A pathological fracture at the

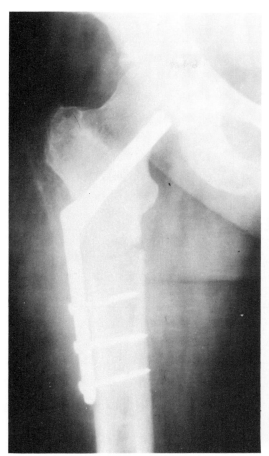

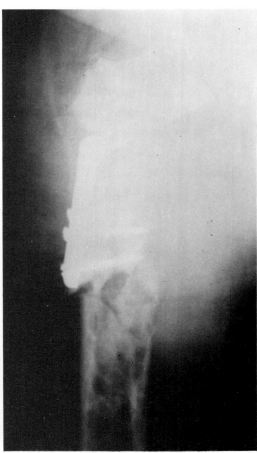

b   c

edge of a plate or intramedullary nail, particularly if the implant has also been fixed with methylmethacrylate, is more difficult to treat than if there was no implant in the bone, and it is extremely difficult to irradiate a metastasis if part of the lesion has been included in a previous field.

Pathological fractures

Although virtually every malignant neoplasm can metastasize to bone, and may be associated with pathological fracture, more than half are secondary to mammary carcinoma (Table 24.1) probably because skeletal metastases from mammary carcinoma occur more commonly than from any other tumour. For example, Fitts and his colleagues (1953) reported an incidence of 47% mammary carcinoma in 2030 patients with skeletal metastases.

The commonest site of pathological fracture is the femur (Table 24.2), but virtually any long bone is at risk.

Primary tumour	No. of patients	No. of fractures
Breast	59	74
Bronchus	13	14
Prostate	10	10
Kidney	4	4
Bladder	2	2
Melanoma	2	2
Stomach	2	2
Thyroid	1	1
Rectum	1	1
Oesophagus	1	1
Bile duct	1	1
Uterus	1	1
Cervix	1	1
Penis	1	1
Squamous cell	1	1
Leukaemia	2	2
Myeloma	7	11
Site unknown	1	1
Total	110	130

Table 24.1 The primary tumour associated with pathological fracture in 110 patients.

Femur	Transcervical	30
	Intertrochanteric	18
	Subtrochanteric	12
	Shaft	26
	Distal	5
Humerus	Proximal	8
	Shaft	28
	Distal	1
Tibia	Shaft	1
Radius	Shaft	1

Table 24.2 Sites of 130 pathological fractures in 110 patients.

Survival	No.
0–3 months	32
4–6 months	5
7–12 months	17
13 + months	15
Mean survival: months	10.1

Table 24.3 Survival following pathological fracture in 69 patients (Galasko, 1974).

The development of a pathological fracture is not necessarily a terminal event, the mean survival after fracture being 10.1 months (Table 24.3). Fifty-four per cent of patients survived for more than three months and 23% for more than one year. The survival is related to the primary tumour, none of our patients with bronchial carcinoma surviving for more than six months, but several of the patients with carcinoma of the breast lived for more than one year after developing a pathological fracture.

There are three aspects to the treatment of pathological fractures.

1 The orthopaedic management;
2 The localized irradiation; and
3 The treatment of the underlying tumour.

The evaluation of a patient with a pathological fracture or impending fracture includes an assessment of the general fitness of the patient, the degree of dissemination, the primary tumour itself, and the presence of other complications, e.g. hypercalcaemia, spinal cord or cauda equina compression. In addition to a careful clinical examination, the evaluation will include appropriate blood tests, X-rays and skeletal scintigrams. If the primary lesion is not known, or there is any uncertainty about the origin of the pathological fracture, a biopsy of the lesion is essential. Usually this can be carried out at the time of surgical stabilization. Biopsy is not an essential part of every internal stabilization, particularly if a closed method of intramedullary fixation is used.

Evaluation of 28 patients with a transcervical femoral fracture showed that no fracture united, irrespective of the method of orthopaedic treatment, probably due to the effect of irradiation on an area where fractures are known to be associated with an impaired vascularity. Furthermore, the failure to unite occurred irrespective of the degree of displacement (Galanko, 1980). This study also showed that primary replacement hemiarthroplasty gave optimum results. All the patients were mobilized within a few days of operation and had no further problems from their proximal femur.

Since the completion of this study, we have treated pathological, transcervical, femoral fractures by replacement arthroplasty. If there are no metastases in the acetabulum or in the remainder of the affected femur, a hemiarthroplasty is carried out. If there is a metastasis in the acetabulum, a total hip replacement is carried out (Fig. 24.3), with curettage of the metastasis, and the defect is filled with methylmethacrylate. If X-rays or scintigraphy show further metastases along the shaft of the affected femur, a long-stemmed hemiarthroplasty or femoral component of a total arthroplasty is used, the length of the stem being sufficient to stabilize all distal metastases in the affected bone.

Unlike transcervical femoral fractures, the majority of patho-

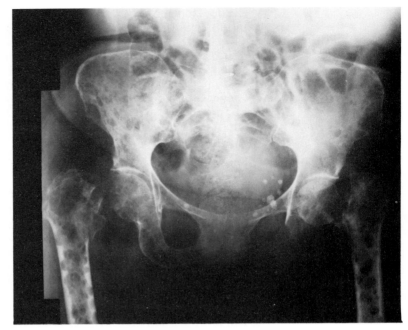

a

logical fractures involving the rest of the femur or tibia united by bone in patients who survived for four or more months, irrespective of the type of treatment. However, internal fixation provided definite advantages over external support. It gave the patient much greater and much more rapid relief of pain; it was associated with easier nursing, more comfortable turning of the patient, and prevention of pressure sores; and it allowed much more rapid mobilization of the patient and earlier discharge from hospital. As with impending fractures, it is essential to adequately stabilize the bone, sufficient for weight-bearing, at the time of surgery. If necessary, the internal fixation must be supplemented by methylmethacrylate (Harrington et al, 1972) even though methylmethacrylate may interfere with callus formation. The use of methylmethacrylate may explain why not all pathological fractures unite by callus. With the adjuvant use of methylmethacrylate, less residual bone is required to support the implant.

The method of internal fixation depends on the site of the fracture. I prefer the use of a Zickel signal-arm nail for subtrochanteric fractures, a dynamic compression screw-plate or Zickel nail for trochanteric fractures, an intramedullary nail for fractures of the shaft of the femur or tibia, Zickel supracondylar nails or angle plates for fractures of the distal femur and plate fixation for fractures of the proximal tibia. Fractures of the metaphysis frequently require methylmethacrylate supplementation.

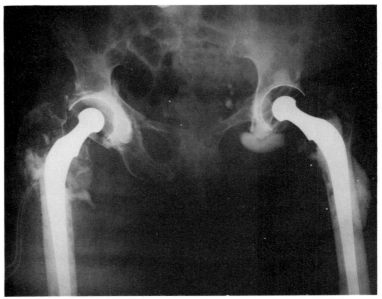

b

Evaluation of 32 pathological fractures of the humerus showed that internal fixation was also of benefit in that it provided the patient with much greater mobility and earlier use of the limb, and more rapid and greater pain relief, but the advantages over conservative treatment were not as marked as with pathological fractures of the lower limb. Fractures of the proximal humerus may require replacement arthroplasty if they cannot be internally fixed. However, the indication for replacement arthroplasty is different to that for transcervical femoral fractures. In the humerus replacement is indicated if it is not possible to stabilize the fracture because of its site or degree of comminution. The vast majority of pathological fractures of the humerus, radius or ulna can be treated by intramedullary nailing. Fractures around the metaphysis may require plate fixation. Where necessary the implant must be supplemented with methylmethacrylate.

Local irradiation is an essential part of treatment. Only one pathological fracture in our series did not receive postoperative radiotherapy. This was associated with progressive destruction of bone and loosening and subsequent breakage of the plate used to stabilize a fracture of the distal femur. The radiation can be delayed until the wound has healed, but this is not essential. The implant did not appear to affect the irradiation, providing megavoltage was used.

Radiotherapy did not interfere with fracture healing, providing the fracture was adequately immobilized (Bonarigo and Rubin, 1967); and fractures of the humeral shaft treated by intramedullary nailing and postoperative radiotherapy healed more rapidly in my series and with greater amounts of callus formation than non-pathological, traumatic fractures at the same site.

Fractures in a patient with malignant disease, but with no evidence of dissemination

Patients with an underlying malignancy may, like any other individual, develop a fracture without a metastasis at the site of fracture. However, if a patient has a past history of mammary carcinoma or any other malignancy, and there is no evidence of dissemination, a biopsy should be taken of the fracture. In some instances this may be the first manifestation of dissemination of the disease even though there has been a long disease-free interval.

The development of a non-pathological fracture, in such a patient, may subsequently be associated with dissemination of the cancer. The author has experience of two patients with mammary carcinoma, one of whom developed a displaced trans-cervical fracture 16 years following mastectomy and the second a fracture-dislocation of a hip 22 years following mastectomy. In both patients there was no evidence of dissemination at the time of the fracture, and histological examination of biopsies taken from the fractured bone ends showed no tumour, yet both patients developed multiple metastases, affecting lung and bone within three months of the fracture.

Spinal instability
Back pain is a frequent symptom in patients with disseminated carcinoma and in 10% is due to spinal instability (Galasko and Sylvester, 1978). Spinal instability can be associated with excru-

Table 24.4 The primary tumour associated with spinal instability.

Tumour	No. of patients
Breast	16
Myeloma	5
Prostate	2
Melanoma	2
Bronchus	1
Parotid	1
Uterus	1
Cervix	1
Vagina	1
Kidney	1
Colon	1
Chondrosarcoma	1
Histiocytoma	1
Cordoma	1
Total	35

Table 24.5
Method of spinal
stabilization.

Harrington rod	5
Harrington rod + sublaminal wiring	1
Banks' rod	26
Luque segmental stabilization: Luque rod	1
Rectangle	2
Total	35

ciating pain, which is mechanical in nature. In the severe form, the patient is only comfortable when lying absolutely still. Any movement, including log-rolling by two or three trained nurses, is associated with great pain, and the patient may not be able to sit, stand or walk because of the pain, even with the use of a spinal jacket. In the milder form, the patient may be relatively free from pain when wearing a rigid spinal orthosis, but movement of the back, turning in bed, sitting or standing is impossible without this support. X-rays show destruction of bone with vertebral collapse to a greater or lesser degree. No discrete fracture can be seen. Nevertheless, spinal instability should be considered the equivalent of a pathological fracture in an appendicular bone, because the pain is due to the instability and not the metastasis. Radiotherapy or chemotherapy will not alleviate the pain. As with pathological fractures of the long bones, immobilization is required for pain relief.

We have treated 35 patients who had spinal instability secondary to spinal metastases. The primary tumours are shown in Table 24.4 and, as with pathological fractures of the skeleton, carcinoma of the breast was the commonest primary tumour. The technique of stabilization used is shown in Table 24.5. Some of the

Figure 24.4
Banks' rod. The
Banks' rod is fixed to
the spine by screws
passing deep to the
spinous process and
into the contralateral
lamina.

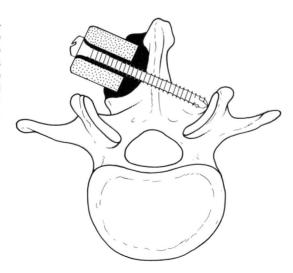

techniques of spinal stabilization are also discussed by John Miles in Chapter 25.

There were three failures. A Banks' rod had to be removed because of infection and one Harrington and one Banks' rod loosened.

The other 32 patients have had relief from their severe pain. One other patient developed an infection which did not require removal of the Banks' rod. She had had relief from pain for over two years, when she required bilateral total hip replacements and a unilateral total shoulder replacement for pathological fractures of both femoral necks and one proximal humerus.

The Harrington rod was designed for the correction of scoliosis

Figure 24.5
Patient with disseminated mammary carcinoma who had spinous instability at the level of D10 and a collapsed 4th lumbar vertebra. Her spine has been stabilized from D7 to the sacrum. A lumbar lordosis has been moulded into the Banks' rod to prevent a postoperative flat back.

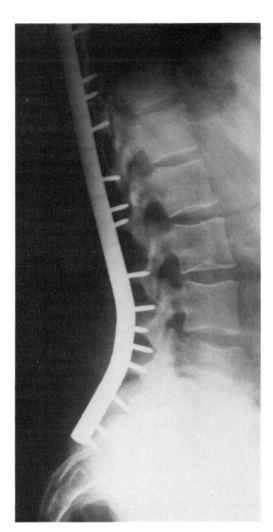

Table 24.6
Associated neurological deficit in patients with spinal instability.

No. of patients	17
No. of patients improved following surgery	12
No. of late cord–cauda equina compression	1
No. of recurrences	2

and is fixed to the spine by hooks at either end of the rod. These hooks eventually loosen. Also in scoliosis a spinal fusion is carried out simultaneously and the spine immobilized in a plaster jacket for six to twelve months while the fusion mass matures. Patients with disseminated carcinoma have a limited life expect-

Figure 24.6
(b–f; see pp. 178–180) Patient with disseminated mammary carcinoma, spinal instability and neurological signs indicating cauda equina compression. (a) and (b) Destruction of L3 with spinal instability. (c) and (d) Radiculogram showing compression of the cauda equina at the level of the metastasis. (e) and (f) Stabilization with a Hartshill rectangle fixed to the spine with sublaminal wires. A lumbar lordosis has been moulded into the implant to allow for comfortable sitting postoperatively.

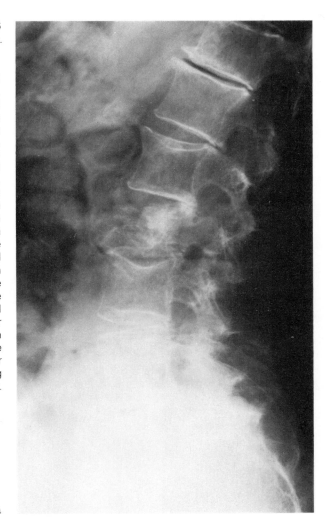

a

---

ancy and it is important to give them maximum quality of life as soon as possible. Therefore, postoperative plaster jackets or spinal orthoses should be avoided.

Methods of spinal stabilization associated with fixation at many levels do not carry this risk of loosening and are preferable for spinal stabilization in this group of patients. The Banks' rod is dependent on screw fixation at multiple levels. The rod is embedded in the gutter between the spinous process and lamina and the screws passed deep to the spinous process into the contralateral lamina (Fig. 24.4). It can be moulded to the shape of the spine, by a special bending instrument.

The Luque rods are cylindrical and can be more easily contoured to the shape of the spine (Fig. 24.5). However, two rods

Figure 24.6b & c

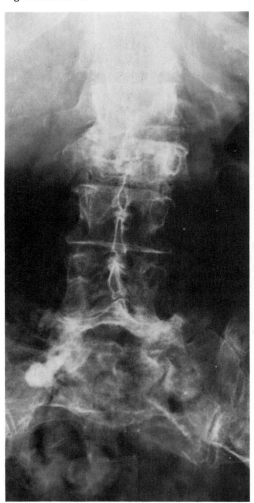
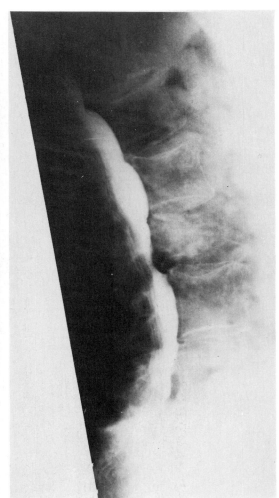

b   c

or a rectangle must be used, the rods being fitted into the gutter between the spinous process and lamina on each side. The rods are fixed to the spine by sublaminal wires, i.e. wires passing under the laminae in the epidural space. Both the Banks' rod and the Luque rod must be fixed to at least two vertebrae above and two vertebrae below the unstable segment.

There was an associated neurological deficit in 17 patients (Table 24.6). These 17 patients did not present because of their cord–cauda equina compression. They presented with pain due to

Figure 24.6d & e

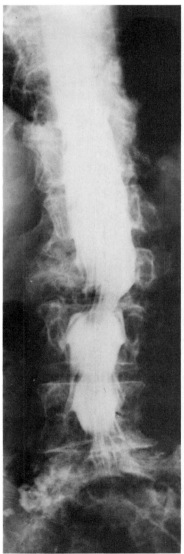
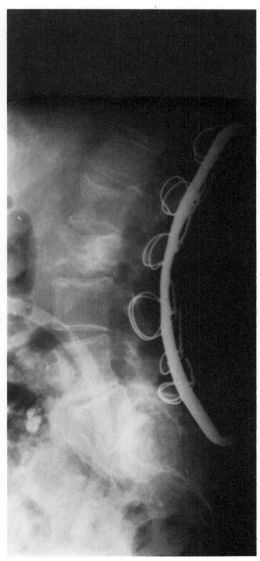

d   e

spinal instability, but evidence of cord or cauda equina compression was found on clinical examination. We routinely carry out a radiculogram prior to spinal stabilization. Irrespective of any clinical evidence of cord–cauda equina compression, the cord–cauda equina is decompressed at the time of stabilization if there is any evidence of compression on the preoperative radiculogram. Both laminae and the spinous process are removed as Banks' or Luque rods provide sufficient stability (Fig. 24.6).

An alternative method of spinal decompression and stabiliza-

Figure 24.6f

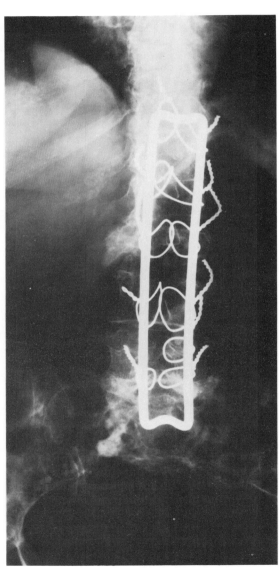

f

Table 24.7
Survival following spinal stabilization in 25 patients (Galasko & Banks, 1985).

Length of survival	No. of patients
0–8 weeks	5
9–16 weeks	7
17–24 weeks	2
25–36 weeks	6
9–12 months	0
13–24 months	4
2–5 years	1

tion is via an anterior approach with excision of the affected vertebral body, decompression of the dural sheath from in front, and subsequent stabilization of the spine using methylmethacrylate (Chapter 25).

As with pathological fractures of the appendicular skeleton postoperative irradiation is an essential part of treatment.

Spinal instability is not a terminal event. Twenty-five of the 35 patients have died. Their mean survival was 32.1 weeks, 15 patients lived for more than three months and 1 patient lived for four years (Table 24.7).

Instability of the cervical spine is rare compared with involvement of the dorsal and lumbar spine, but occurs occasionally. The principle of treatment is the same, namely spinal stabilization, and decompression if there is any evidence of cord compression, followed by radiotherapy.

Conclusions

1 The development of an impending fracture, pathological fracture or spinal instability is not necessarily a terminal event.
2 These lesions are associated with severe pain.
3 The aims of treatment are to alleviate pain and restore mobility and use of the affected limb or spine.
4 With the exception of pathological transcervical femoral fractures, this is best achieved by internal stabilization.
5 The type of stabilization depends on the site of the lesion.
6 If the stabilization is not adequate to provide unsupported use of the limb, it should be supplemented by methylmethacrylate.
7 Postoperative radiotherapy is an essential part of the treatment.
8 The underlying tumour can be treated by hormonal therapy or chemotherapy, where indicated.
9 Before these lesions are treated the patient must be carefully evaluated to determine the degree of dissemination of the cancer, particularly for any other areas of involvement in the affected bone, as this may influence the type of stabilization.
10 Optimum treatment of these lesions requires major surgery,

which probably should not be carried out if the patient is terminal. If the patient has only a few days to live we make them comfortable, and immobilize the fracture or unstable spine with some form of suitable support. However, if in our opinion, the patient is likely to survive for at least three to four weeks, major surgery to palliate the severe symptoms secondary to fractures and spinal instability is indicated.

Controversies and Future Developments

• Is expensive surgery justified in patients with so poor a prognosis?
• The possibility of predicting bone metastases and using prophylactic irradiation to prevent the distressing effects.

Further reading

Banks, A.J. & Dervin, E. (1980) A simple method for the stabilisation of malignant spine. *Engineering in Medicine*, 9, 81–83.

Bonarigo, B.C. & Rubin, P. (1967) Non-union of pathologic fracture after radiation therapy. *Radiology*, 88, 889–898.

Campbell, C.J. (1967) In: *Palliative Care of the Cancer Patient*, ed. Hickey, R.C. Boston: Little, Brown & Co.

Edelstyn, G.A., Gillespie, P.J. & Grebbell, F.S. (1967) The radiological demonstration of osseous metastases. Experimental observations. *Clin. Radiol.*, 18, 158–162.

Fidler, M. (1973) Prophylactic internal fixation of secondary neoplastic deposits in long bones. *Br. Med. J.*, 1, 341–343.

Fitts, W.T., Roberts, B. & Ravdin, I.S. (1953) Fractures in metastatic carcinoma. *Am. J. Surg.*, 85, 282–287.

Galasko, C.S.B. (1974) Pathological fractures secondary to metastatic cancer. *J. Royal Coll. Surg. Edin.*, 19, 351–362.

Galasko, C.S.B. (1980) The management of skeletal metastases. *J. Royal Coll. Surg. Edin.*, 25, 143–161.

Galasko, C.S.B. & Banks, A.J. (1985) The stabilisation of skeletal metastases. In: *Treatment of Metastasis: Problems and Prospects*, ed. Hellmann, K. & Eccles, S.A. London: Taylor & Francis.

Galasko, C.S.B. & Sylvester, B.S. (1978) Back pain in patients treated for malignant tumours. *Clin. Oncol.*, 4, 273–283.

Harrington, K.D., Johnston, J.O., Turner, R.H. & Green, D.L. (1972) The use of methylmethacrylate as an adjunct in the internal fixation of malignant neoplastic fractures. *J. Bone Joint Surg.*, 54-A, 1665–1676.

Zickel, R.E. & Mouradian, W.H. (1976) Intramedullary fixation of pathological fractures and lesions of the subtrochanteric region of the femur. *J. Bone Joint Surg.*, 58-A, 1061–1066.

25 Vertebral Metastases

John Miles

The fact that the vertebrae contain red marrow makes them preferred sites for metastases. By virtue of the substantial incidence, spinal metastases from carcinoma from the breast generate considerable problems for several medical and surgical disciplines: not only those involved wth the primary treatment of the breast cancer (general surgery, oncology, radiotherapy) but also those specialties devoted specifically to the spine (orthopaedics, physical medicine) or spinal cord (neurosurgery, neurology).

The true incidence of spinal metastases in the community is not recorded but has been estimated by this author to be as much as 1 in 20 000. The relative proportion of breast metastases amongst all spinal metastases presenting to a District General Hospital has been recorded as 28%, being second only in frequency to that of carcinoma of the lung (33%).

Most spinal carcinoma metastases occur in the vertebral bodies and although presentation appears to be more commonly caused by thoracic deposits, in fact the distribution throughout the spine is relatively even (Torma, 1957). Deposits within the extradural space do occur in isolation, but much more commonly they arise from deposits in the bone of the vertebrae.

Clinical features

Pain is the commonest and earliest symptom (Brice and McKissock, 1965). The most common site for the pain is interscapular, with later radiculopathic propagation. It tends to precede neurological symptoms by months even though, during this period, it is rare for the true pathology to be recognized. The pain may be typical for bone malignancy, being relatively constant, particularly at night, and is presumably due to periosteal distension by the expanding mass. Sometimes the pain reflects spinal instability by being worse on movement and weight-bearing and only being relieved by splintage or recumbency. Galasko and Sylvester found instability pain in 3 out of 33 patients, but the true incidence seems to be much higher once the significance of instability is recognized. Radiculopathic pain may be due to root compression by soft tumour mass but is more likely to be due to instability, collapse or angulation.

The radiculopathic symptoms may take the form of paraesthesiae, anaesthesia, wasting, weakness and loss of reflexes, and it is when these features occur in the arms and legs that they become recognized. More commonly, however, the spinal cord, down as far as L2, is compressed by deposits. The symptoms then are of the gradual onset of spastic weakness of the legs (paraparesis) sometimes with numbness and clumsiness of gait and followed after a variable interval by retention of urine and constipation. Rarely, this syndrome occurs rapidly and then there is usually evidence of collapse of a vertebral body.

Percussion over the vertebral bodies at the level of back pain is a valuable monoeuvre as pain is commonly aggravated and may radiate in a radiculopathic manner.

Investigations

Radiographs of the suspected spine are essential and will often prove sufficient to reveal the deposits. The lesions are most commonly lytic with evidence of collapse (Fig. 25.1a). The changes may, however, be more subtle and demand careful scrutiny (Fig. 25.1b). Chest radiographs are necessary to assess the dissemination of carcinomatosis.

Isotope bone scanning may be necessary when plain radiographs fail to reveal a lesion or to assess the degree of other bony involvement (Fig. 25.2).

Figure 25.1 (a) Radiograph showing vertebral body collapse (arrowed) due to lytic metastasis. (b) Anteroposterior radiograph showing loss of pedicular outline (arrowed) without collapse.

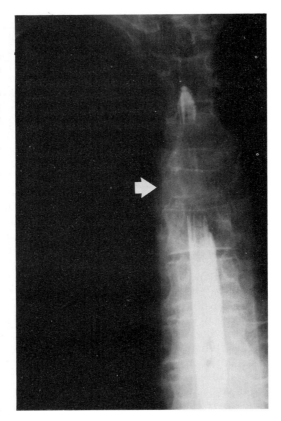

a

Myelography is indicated if surgery is being considered for either pain or neurological features. It is better performed in a unit with neurosurgical facilities so that urgent decompression can be undertaken should neurological deterioration occur as a result of the hydrodynamic changes associated with loss of CSF during or after lumbar puncture. CT scanning delineates focal and metastatic deposits well but is still not always available. CT screening for additional deposits would seem to be an unjustified waste of valuable scanning facilities. Magnetic Resonance Imaging very beautifully illustrates local and multiple deposits in the vertebrae but at the moment it is even less readily available.

Treatment

General
Pituitary destruction in the management of widespread pain due to advanced carcinomatosis is definitely a viable option. This manoeuvre may relieve bone pain independent of any hormonal effect it exerts upon the tumour; the mechanism is unknown.

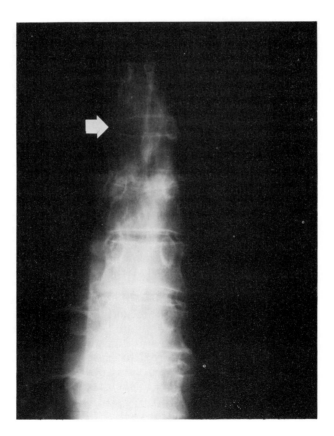

b

Figure 25.2
Isotope bone scan
showing multiple
vertebral areas of
increased uptake due
to metastic cancer.

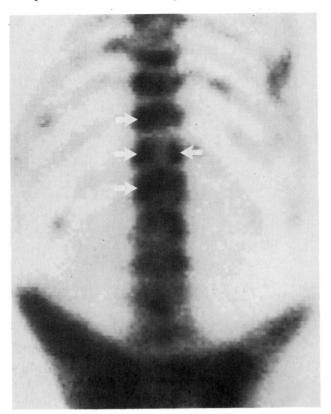

Figure 25.2
Isotope bone scan showing multiple vertebral areas of increased uptake due to metastic cancer.

Destruction of the pituitary may be carried out surgically, the transphenoidal route being preferable, or by alcohol injection transphenoretally. Since hypophysectomy is a suitable procedure for second-line hormone therapy it is therefore worth considering its use at an earlier stage in patients with painful bony metastases and possibly combining second-line hormone therapy and pain relief by hypophysectomy.

Local treatment
Focal radiotherapy can undoubtedly relieve pain due to spinal metastases, although it is not necessarily immediate and sometimes can be associated with a major 'flare effect' with exacerbation of the pain and possibly even the neurological deficit. In general, it is reserved for deposits without clinical or radiological evidence of instability and when there is limited evidence of myelographic threat to the cord or cauda equina.

A steroid cover, using large doses of dexamethasone, is an advisable prelude to such treatment. No authoritative comparison of radiotherapy with surgical or combined surgical and radiotherapy programmes has been made. When neurological features have developed and myelography reveals evidence of compression, the common surgical management has been to perform at the earliest opportunity an exploratory and decompressive laminectomy. In addition to obtaining histological diagnosis and excluding more benign conditions, it has been used to protect neurological function and, by some, to relieve root pain. As the routine management it is probably no longer justified.

Histological identification of the tissue involved is now achievable by lesser procedures than laminectomy, such as needle/cannula biopsy.

The results of laminectomy with regard to neurological deterioration have been clearly outlined (Findlay, 1984). There can be no doubt but that instability is aggravated by laminectomy.

Recognition of the problem of instability of the spine affected by metastases led Scoville et al (1967) to the use of acrylic, initially posteriorly with lattice reinforcement with stainless

Figure 25.3
(a) Anterior and posterior bony fusion for metastases of the cervical spine.
(b): overleaf.

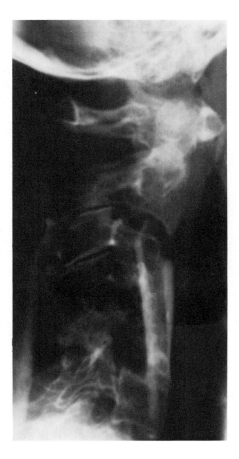

steel wire, but also anteriorly with replacement of the diseased vertebral body.

As the weight-bearing in the spine runs primarily through the vertebral bodies and since they are most frequently involved with metastases, the ideal approach would appear to be anteriorly. Certainly in the neck, access from in front is not difficult and the body or bodies can be totally replaced by synthetic prostheses or by a bone graft. If bone is used, then some form of additional fixation or stabilization is necessary either by prolonged (3 months) external bracing (Fig. 25.3a) or, more appropriately in the context of advanced cancer, by internal fixation using some form of plate or rod (Fig. 25.3b).

As for the rest of the spine, anterior access is much more difficult, involving special and unusual experience or combined surgery. It is also much more demanding of the patient and would seem applicable only when the natural history of the malignancy has taken an unusually indolent course. Harrington (1981) revealed that major anterior surgery, with vertebral body

Figure 25.3
(b) Anterior bony fusion after vertebral body replacement with internal fixation using a stainless steel bar and screws.

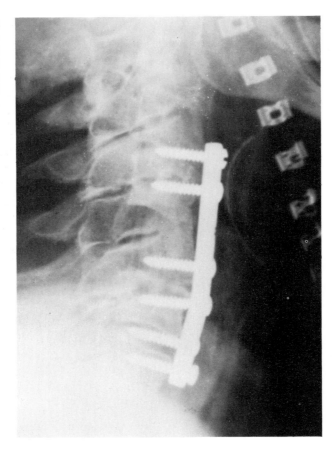

replacement by acrylic together with rod fixation, was both possible and remarkably effective with regard to survival and quality of neurological restitution. This approach can also involve the use of bone grafting of the resected body or bodies (Fig. 25.4) and, again, either external bracing or internal rod fixation can be used. The latter is particularly applicable if laminectomy has already been undertaken.

Suitable patients, with the special qualities already mentioned, would seem to be relatively infrequent. Most patients with vertebral deposits of disseminated carcinoma from the breast appear to have too advanced disease to tolerate such major surgery.

Banks et al (1985) applied themselves to designing an internal fixation bar that could be applied using the posterior approach and this has proved to be very effective in relieving pain and to be of some value in easing neurological deficit.

The comparative virtues of the technique, together with the technical details, are discussed by Banks et al (1985). Essentially,

Figure 25.4
Lateral radiograph of the thoracic spine showing an anterior transthoracic vertebral body resection with bone graft (arrowed).

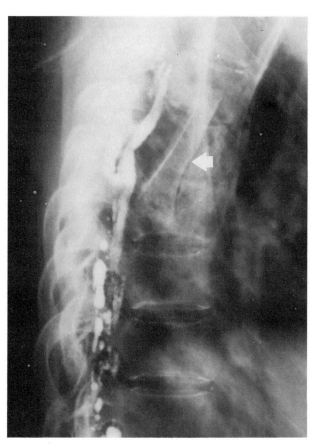

a multiperforated but exceedingly strong, square section, stainless steel rod is secured into the posterior vertebral arches so that the screws pass into the base of the spinous processes in the line of the opposite lamina. A thin layer of acrylic is insinuated between the suitably formed rod and the underlying vertebrae and while this is still maleable, the screws are finally screwed home. Additional wiring through holes and around laminae, or through spinous processes, can also be incorporated when there is any concern over fixation.

The technique allows exploratory or decompressive laminectomy if this is desired, and does not preclude the use of postoperative radiotherapy. It is indicated if instability pain is present, when neurological deficit appears related to instability, and if laminectomy is to be undertaken.

Conclusions

1 In the context of known carcinoma from the breast, vertebral pain should be investigated by plain radiographs and radioisotope scanning.

2 A needle biopsy may obviate the need for surgical exploration when the diagnosis is not apparent.

3 Focal radiotherapy may prove very successful in relieving the 'bone' pain.

4 A relatively easy posterior surgical technique exists which is probably applicable to metastatic deposits at any segment of the spine. Surgery is indicated once neurological features develop and there is myelographic evidence of compression.

5 Stabilization of an affected segment of the spine may be justified purely because of pain, even that involved in nursing an already bedridden patient.

Further reading

Banks, A.J., Dervin, E. & Miles, J.B. (1985) Surgical treatment of instability in metastatic disease of the spine. In: *Persistent Pain*, Vol. V, ed. Lipton, S. & Miles, J.B. London: Academic Press.

Brice, J. & McKissock, W.S. (1965) Surgical treatment of malignant extradural spinal tumours. *Br. Med. J., (1)*, 1341–1344.

Findlay, G.F.G. (1984) Adverse effects of the management of malignant spinal cord compression. *J. Neurol. Neurosurg. Psychiat.*, 47, 761–768.

Harrington, K. (1981) The use of methyl-methacrylate for vertebral bony replacement and anterior stabilisation of pathological fracture dislocations of the spine due to metastic malignant disease. *J. Bone Joint Surg., 63a*, 36–46.

Kakulas, B.A., Harper, C.G., Shibasaki, K. & Bedbrook, G.M. (1980) Vertebral metastases and spinal cord compression. *Clin. Exp. Neurol.*, *15*, 98–113.

Miles, J.B., Banks, J., Dervin, E. & Noori, Z. (1984) Stabilisation of the spine affected by malignancy. *J. Neurol. Neurosurg. Psychiat.*, 47, 897–904.

Miles, J.B. (1984) Pituitary destruction for the relief of pain. In: *A Textbook of Pain*. ed. Wall, P.D. & Melzack, R. pp. 656–665. London: Churchill Livingstone.

Scoville, W.B., Palmer, A.H., Samra, K. & Chong, G. (1967) The use of acrylic plastic for vertebral replacement or fixation on metastatic disease of the spine. *J. Neurosurg.*, *27*, 274–279.

Torma, T. (1957) Malignant tumours of the spine and the spinal extradural space. A study based on 250 histologically verified cases. *Acta, Chirurg, Scand., Suppl. 225*, 9–176.

26 Pleural Effusions and Breathlessness

Michael Williams

The development of a malignant pleural effusion as a sequel of metastatic breast cancer is a frequent finding in the postmastectomy follow-up clinic. Carcinoma of the breast most commonly recurs locally in the draining axillary lymph nodes or mastectomy flap, with the axial skeleton being the most common site for the initial presentation of distant metastases. However, the lung parenchyma, pleura and mediastinal lymph nodes are all common sites in which distant metastases first appear. In patients undergoing treatment for advanced disease, approximately 50% will develop an effusion at some stage in their disease (Frachia et al, 1970).

The pleural space when unaffected by disease contains no more than 5–20 ml of fluid. This fluid is formed by the parietal and absorbed by the visceral pleura. It has a low protein content and a similar electrolyte constitution to interstitial fluid. There is a continuous flux of fluid throughout the pleural space and an equilibrium is set up between hydrostatic and osmotic forces together with lymphatic drainage, so that under normal circumstances the volume of fluid within the space remains constant. When this equilibrium is disturbed by disease, fluid collects and an effusion develops.

The factors involved in the formation of an effusion can be divided into three main categories:

Firstly, and most commonly, direct infiltration of the pleura by malignant cells produces malignant plaques with an exudate of fluid developing in the pleural cavity in response to increased capillary permeability. Direct invasion of pleural vessels by tumour may also produce an haemorrhagic effusion.

Secondly, lymphatic blockage by malignant involvement of mediastinal or hilar lymph nodes, impairs lymphatic drainage, so increasing capillary pressure producing an accumulation of fluid in the pleural space. Lymphatic enlargement may also result in bronchial obstruction, producing secondary infection distally and a reactive effusion.

Finally, and perhaps least commonly, venous obstruction by malignant growth increases capillary pressure as a direct result of increasing venous back pressure and results in the formation of an effusion.

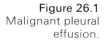

Figure 26.1
Malignant pleural
effusion.

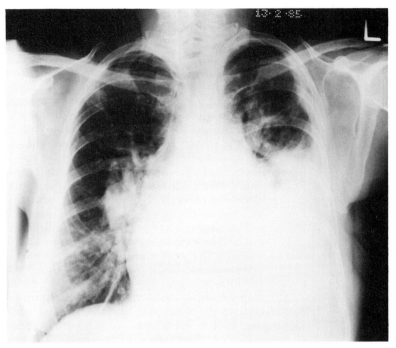

Clinical presentation, assessment and treatment

In all cases the presence of disseminated malignancy must be differentiated from other benign causes of effusion. However, it is noteworthy that, in the great majority of patients presenting with a pulmonary effusion and a previous history of breast carcinoma, disseminated malignancy is implicated.

A malignant effusion (Fig. 26.1) may present asymptomatically or the patient may complain of increasing breathlessness with classic symptoms and signs.

The diagnosis is made by taking a history and performing a clinical examination with particular reference to other likely signs of disseminated malignant disease. The diagnosis is confirmed radiologically. A history of recent respiratory tract infection or previous episodes of cardiac failure may suggest these two common benign differential diagnoses. Symptomatic malignant effusions often present with rapidly increasing dyspnoea and, in many cases, other symptoms attributable to metastatic disease. Clinical signs are often absent with small effusions, but as fluid collects a combination of dullness to percussion and diminished breath sounds develops. When unilateral, the effusion often presents on the same side as the previous mastectomy, and the apex beat is displaced away from the affected side.

In all patients further investigations are performed to establish the extent of disease. These include haematological tests with a full blood count, erythrocyte sedimentation rate and liver function tests. A limited skeletal survey is required to exclude concomitant bone metastases or to act as a base line, if these are present, in order to assess later response to treatment. Hepatic and brain scans are performed only when clinically indicated. A chest X-ray should include lateral views since small effusions are more easily seen in the dependent posterior gutter.

In the presence of indisputable extrathoracic metastatic disease it is not always necessary to pursue the cause of a small asymptomatic effusion. This can be treated expectantly, using extra thoracic disease to assess any response to systemic treatment. Where there is no other sign of distant disease, the fluid must be examined cytologically and microbiologically in an attempt to confirm the suspected diagnosis of metastatic disease.

The therapeutic aspiration of a pulmonary effusion is carried out under strict asepsis. The patient should be kept comfortable through the procedure by positioning her seated with arms and head supported on a raised couch or over the back of a chair. Local anaesthetic is then injected into all layers at the site of aspiration. An Abrams needle is then inserted into the pleural cavity to obtain at least 50 ml of aspirate to perform the diagnostic investigations. Several pleural biopsies should be taken at the same time for histological examination. This can be conveniently achieved using the same Abrams needle. Complete aspiration of the effusion is possible using this needle, however in large effusions it is often less traumatic to insert an indwelling chest drain with an underwater seal. In addition to allowing more complete aspiration of the pleural space, this also enables the fluid to be withdrawn in aliquots so preventing any added complications or discomfort for the patient.

Pleural fluid may appear straw-coloured, clear or blood-stained. In the presence of an empyema, the effusion will be purulent, and opalescent when due to a chylothorax. After exclusion of accidental haemorrhage at the time of aspiration, red blood counts above 100 000 cells per ml of fluid are diagnostic of infarction, trauma or malignancy. Biochemical tests may help to establish the diagnosis in difficult cases. These include measurement of the specific gravity, protein content, and lactate dehydrogenase level of the aspirated fluid. Malignant exudates frequently have a specific gravity above 1016, with a protein content above 30 g/litre and a lactate dehydrogenase content above 200 I.U./ml. Unfortunately all these investigations are by no means entirely specific. When cytological examination is performed, malignant cells may be seen when the pleura is invaded by tumour. In cases of malignant effusion without direct invasion of pleura, these cells will not be present in the aspirate. Unfortunately, this, again, is not entirely specific and also requires the attentions of an expert cytologist. False-negative rates of around 40% have been recorded when the diagnosis is made on cytology alone (Martinez-Vea et al, 1982). The importance of a variety of tumour markers to increase the discrimination between benign and malignant effusions has been assessed by several investigators (Couch, 1981). The results are conflicting but abnormally high CEA, HCG and orosomucoid levels in serous effusions have been suggested as being useful adjuncts to cytological examination. Recently, the development of monoclonal antibody technology has provided another method by which malignant cells can be identified by their tumour-specific antigens (Epenetos et al, 1982).

A sample of aspirate is sent to the microbiology laboratory for microscopy, culture and sensitivity. These tests are also often disappointing due to the inevitable delays in samples reaching the laboratory or to the frequent use of antibiotics prior to aspiration when infection is suspected.

Management of recurrent effusions

Patients with malignant effusions from carcinoma of the breast are incurable and so recurrence is often a problem. The survival in some cases may be many months or years and so treatment in these patients should be aimed not only at relieving symptoms at presentation, but should also attempt to reduce the chance of any recurrence. In one series of 127 patients with malignant effusions from breast cancer the median survival was six months (Raja and Kardinal, 1981). Anderson et al in 1974 reported disappointing results after the use of thoracocentesis alone. He studied 94 patients in whom there was a 97% recurrence rate one month after treatment by thoracocentesis only. In addition, these recurrences were usually associated with symptoms and often required further therapy.

Drainage by closed-tube thoracocentesis with continuous suction applied to the underwater seal, so encouraging pleural surfaces to adhere, reduces recurrence rates. However, the best results have been obtained with the insertion of a sclerosant agent into the pleural space immediately following complete aspiration of the fluid. Several different agents have been used for this purpose. These include radioisotopes, tetracycline, corynebacterium parvum, mepacrine, bleomycin, nitrogen mustard and thiotepa. Systemic analgesia, or the addition of a local anaesthetic to the sclerosant, is necessary as the associated pleurisy is frequently painful. After allowing the effusion to drain completely the tube is clamped and disconnected. A suitable syringe, which fits tightly into the disconnected drain, is filled with sclerosant and connected. The tube is unclamped and the sclerosant is injected slowly. The tube is then reclamped, the syringe removed, and the drain reconnected to the underwater seal. The patient is then asked to lie supine while the end of the bed is raised, her position being alternated from side to side every 30 minutes. By these manoeuvres the sclerosant should reach all quarters of the pleural cavity. After this has been completed, the drainage tube is again unclamped and the sclerosant allowed to drain. Suction may now be applied to the underwater seal if deemed necessary. The chest drain is left in situ to allow complete drainage of all sclerosant and is then removed. A chest X-ray is always obtained after drainage to ensure that all fluid has been withdrawn and the lung is well expanded.

Few complications are associated with thoracocentesis; however, if a large effusion is drained too quickly the rapid re-expansion of the lung may produce pulmonary oedema. In large effusions, therefore, it is prudent to drain the fluid in aliquots by clamping and unclamping the tube. Very rarely, pleural puncture may cause vagal inhibition and shock, and so adequate analgesia is always required to prevent this complication. Rapid and frequent removal of fluid with a high protein content may on occasion produce hypoproteinaemia. Air embolus and empyema are also rare complications. Apart from thoracocentesis for symptomatic reasons and to confirm the diagnosis, additional systemic treatments are implemented. Endocrine therapies employing oophorectomy in the premenopausal patient or tamoxifen in the postmenopausal patient, will produce temporary regression or stabilization of disease in approximately 30% of cases.

Assessment of Response to Treatment
The UICC guidelines for the objective assessment of a response to treatment in advanced breast cancer excludes patients where pleural effusions are the only site of distant disease (Hayward et al, 1977). The majority of patients will, however, have other measurable sites of metastatic disease where an assessment of a response to treatment can be made to aid clinical management. Additional local treatments such as radiotherapy may be required to reduce the tumour bulk in mediastinal lymph nodes which are causing obstruction to lymphatic return, resulting in effusion. More aggressive local measures, including operative pleurectomy in those patients refractory to thoracocentesis, have been attempted to control recurrent symptoms from effusions in other types of malignancy. These techniques are not applicable in metastatic breast cancer.

Conclusions
The distressing breathlessness, associated with a pulmonary effusion in advanced breast cancer, is easily remediable with little cost to the patient. In those unresponsive to systemic treatments and with short life expectancy thoracocentesis alone may be adequate to control symptoms until death results from progressive metastatic disease. In others an attempt should be made to prevent recurrence of symptoms and many agents have been employed for this purpose. Intrapleural tetracycline has been shown to be an effective sclerosant with few side-effects, and is the agent of choice in our department at the present time.

Other causes of breathlessness associated with metastatic disease

Intrapulmonary involvement by tumour in the advanced breast cancer patient presents as either solitary or multiple nodules throughout the lung fields or, alternatively, as a diffuse infiltration of the intrapulmonary lymphatics, i.e. carcinomatous lymphangitis. Solitary nodules rarely cause respiratory embarrassment but, when multiple and extensive, they may lead to sufficient loss of effective lung volume to cause breathlessness. Lymphangitis carcinomatosa, however, is frequently associated with severe respiratory impairment. Secondary infection often accompanies this condition and X-ray appearances are difficult to differentiate in some instances from those of pulmonary oedema from other causes. Oral steroids with the addition of broncodilators and broad-spectrum antibiotics may provide a degree of palliation in some patients. Cytotoxic therapy may also in some cases result in dramatic symptomatic improvement and breathlessness, due to lymphangitis of the lung, is a strong indication for the need of this therapy.

References

Anderson, C.B., Philpott, G.W. & Ferguson, T.B. (1974) The treatment of malignant pleural effusions. *Cancer*, *33*, 916–922.

Couch, W.D. (1981) Combined effusion fluid tumor marker assay, carcinoembryonic antigen (CEA) and human chorionic gonadotrophin (HCG) in the detection of malignant tumors. *Cancer*, *48 (11)*, 2475–2479.

Epenetos, A.A., Canti, G., Taylor-Papadimitriou, J., Curling, M. & Bodomer, W.F. (1982) Use of two epithelium-specific monoclonal antibodies for diagnosis of malignancy in serious effusions. *Lancet, ii*, 1004–1006.

Frachia, A.A., Knapper, W.H., Carey, J.T. & Farrow, J.H. (1970) Intra pleural chemotherapy for effusion from metastatic breast cancer. *Cancer*, *26*, 626–629.

Hayward, J.L., Carbonne, P.P., Henson, J.C. et al (1977) Assessment of response to therapy in advanced breast cancer. *Cancer*, *39*, 1289–1293.

Martinez-Vea, A., Gatell, J.M., Segura, F. et al (1982) Diagnostic value of tumoral markers in serious effusions. Carcinoembryonic antigen; alpha 1-acidglycoprotein, alpha-fetoprotein, phosphohexose isomerase, beta-2 microglobulin. *Cancer*, *50 (9)*, 1783–1788.

Raju, R.N. & Kardinal, C.G. (1981) Pleural effusion in breast carcinoma: analysis of 122 cases. *Cancer*, *48 (11)*, 2524–2527.

27 Ascites

Michael Kettlewell and Patricia Clarke

Malignant ascites is a distressing affliction affecting the minority of patients with advanced disease. Accumulation of fluid within the peritoneum usually requires a large intra-abdominal tumour load, but not all cases with such a load will develop ascites. Nevertheless, ascites nearly always occurs in the final months of the patient's life, so treatment is aimed at relief without the addition of a major therapeutic burden.

It is commonly supposed that neoplastic and inflammatory ascites is an exudate, in contrast to cirrhotic ascites, which is a transudate. This characterization is almost certainly an oversimplification for there are all too few data on the chemical composition of malignant ascites and its mechanism of production.

In a proportion of patients, the mechanism for accumulating ascites appears similar to that in patients with cirrhosis. The evidence for this is twofold; firstly, the protein content and characteristics of the ascites is often similar to that from cirrhotics and is just as variable (Henderson et al, 1980). Secondly, patients often respond to the same diuretic regimen as patients with portal hypertension (Greenway et al, 1982). The mechanism for ascites in cirrhosis is fairly well understood. The primary mechanism is sodium and water retention induced by hyperaldosteronism; in the case of cirrhosis this is produced not only by a reduced renal plasma flow, but also by decreased hepatic degradation of aldosterone. The sodium and water retention expands the extracellular fluid compartment, which is then sequestered within the peritoneum because of the portal venous hypertension. Partial lymphatic obstruction within the liver and porta hepatis may also be contributory. The degree of lymphatic obstruction may account for the variations in protein content of the ascites, which is generally lower than that of plasma. Hyperaldosteronism probably exists in patients with malignant ascites but, with the exception of patients who have a large hepatic tumour load, decreased hepatic degradation of aldosterone and portal hypertension cannot be important mechanisms. This means that the tumour must exert a more subtle and direct effect upon fluid secretion and absorption by the peritoneum, which remains susceptible to aldosterone antagonists.

Lymphatic obstruction is fairly common because of infiltration of the intestinal mesentery by carcinoma as well as by lymph-node metastases which may ultimately obstruct the cisterna chyli. Initially, the ascites will be clear but rich in lymphocytes and plasma cells and with a relatively high plasma-protein concentration. However, as the lymphatic obstruction becomes more complete, the fluid becomes more chylous which is an unusual occurrence in clinical practice.

The ascites in some patients is viscid and even mucoid. In these circumstances the ascites is often loculated. This type is clearly a secretory product of the malignant cells and is usually associated with mucous-secreting carcinomas of the ovary and gastrointestinal tract, but, rarely, it may occur from breast metastases. Commoner forms of ascites may also have a secretory component to their aetiology, particularly when the tumour is from secretory epithelium, such as the breast, but cellular secretion is difficult to study and prove in clinical practice.

Ascites is sometimes blood-stained and contains fibrin clots, and in such cases the tumour deposits on the peritoneum induce an inflammatory reaction. The peritoneal surface becomes injected, thickened, haemorrhagic, and contains copious new blood vessels. It is difficult not to assume, in these circumstances, that the tumour is producing the inflammatory response which in turn produces an exudative ascites, rather like tuberculosis, which is rich in protein, fibrin and acute inflammatory cells.

Clearly, there are different potential mechanisms involved in the production of malignant ascites and in any individual case the mechanism which predominates may differ. This, in turn, makes treatment somewhat unpredictable, particularly as similar morphological types of tumour may produce ascites by different mechanisms. An example of the unpredictable nature of tumours is that some 20% of patients with malignant ascites do not give a diagnostic yield of malignant cells, even from a generous paracentesis. Other tumours of the same type, by contrast, exfoliate myriads of malignant cells into the ascitic fluid. The difference in biological behaviour does not correlate with metastasis formation (Tarin et al, 1984) and therefore may imply differences in mechanism for ascites production.

Symptoms from malignant ascites

Increasing abdominal girth, and the weight of fluid, produce discomfort and distress. The discomfort depends partly on the rate of accumulation of the ascites and partly on its volume. Rapid accumulation produces disproportionate discomfort by stretching the abdominal wall, in contrast to more gradual accumulation which allows the abdominal wall to accommodate a large volume. Tissue laxity may also be facilitated by changes in the hepatic metabolism of oestrogen and progesterone.

Gross ascites gives a feeling of permanent pregnancy and the victim feels cumbersome. The obvious distortion is apparent to friends and neighbours and may excite comment from the tactless. Clothes that fit and are comfortable become difficult. Movement and agility are also greatly reduced.

Pain is seldom a major clinical problem except after paracentesis in patients with inflammatory ascites when the friction of the inflamed parietal and visceral peritoneum, in contact with each other, produces peritonism and occasionally partial obstruction.

Dyspnoea is often an important distressing consequence of ascites. The diaphragm becomes progressively raised and splinted. The rise in intra-abdominal pressure may be sufficient to raise intrathoracic pressure to the point of interfering with venous return to the heart. Cardiac failure may then complicate the clinical picture. Reduced ventilation will also promote sputum retention, respiratory-tract infections and bronchopneumonia.

Large amounts of plasma protein become sequestered in the peritoneal cavity and are therefore lost to the effective plasma-protein pool. This loss is greatly accentuated when the ascites is tapped repeatedly. Frequent paracentesis may even exceed the liver's capacity to synthesize albumin, particularly in the face of the higher metabolic demands caused by the tumour. Hypoalbuminaemia leads to peripheral oedema which, in turn, is exacerbated by salt and water retention and the pressure of the ascites on the vena cava. Grossly swollen ankles and calves add to the distress of the dying. Malnutrition is therefore a common accompaniment of ascites, because of the anorexia and hypermetabolism induced by the tumour and because of the loss of albumin. Repeated paracentesis contributes to the malnutrition and consequent muscle wasting and weakness which accentuates the lethargy and apathy associated with terminal malignancy.

Treatment of malignant ascites

1 *Paracentesis*

Repeated and even frequent paracentesis was the only reliable method of relieving ascites, but it is to be deprecated for several reasons. Firstly, it is an uncomfortable procedure, particularly when performed by inexperienced house staff—the people most often deputed to perform the procedure. Secondly, the patient needs to spend several periods of a few days in hospital when every hour spent at home is important and precious. Thirdly, repeated paracentesis hastens malnutrition and hypoalbuminaemia, whose consequences have already been discussed.

Furthermore, paracentesis usually gives imperfect control of the ascites. When tapped dry, patients may suffer pain for a few days and they also clearly suffer from the ascites in the days and weeks before paracentesis. Repeated abdominal puncture also often leads to implantation metastases in the trochar track.

Nevertheless, paracentesis still has a useful role, usually as the first procedure. Occasionally, patients inexplicably do not reaccumulate the peritoneal fluid even without the addition of cytotoxic agents. This response is unpredictable but makes the procedure particularly appropriate when the cause of the ascites is uncertain and cytological examination of the fluid or laparoscopy is necessary.

2 *Chemotherapy*

Patients are usually receiving systemic therapy for secondary breast cancer (Chapter 18). Ascites, as a complication of breast cancer, is sufficiently uncommon for there to be no convincing studies upon the efficacy of either systemic or intraperitoneal chemotherapy.

Several cytotoxic agents have been tried intraperitonealy: thiotepa at 0.8 mg/kg as a bolus dose at the end of paracentesis may be beneficial (Anderson, 1968). Bleomycin and 5-fluoroura-acil have also been used but appear to confer no additional advantage and bleomycin may be painful (Trotter et al, 1979). Our preference is to use intracavity thiotepa after the first paracentesis, in combination with diuretic therapy, as the first-line of treatment. But repeated intracavity cytotoxic instillations have little therapeutic value.

3 *Diuretic therapy*

The majority of cirrhotics with ascites are successfully treated by salt restriction, protein supplementation, spironolactone treatment, and a loop diuretic. Similar treatment, without the burden of salt restriction, has been shown to be effective, not only in reducing the reaccumulation of ascites after paracentesis, but also in reducing the volume of ascites once established. The response to this kind of therapy suggests that, at least in some patients, the genesis of the ascites is similar in patients with intraperitoneal malignancy and cirrhosis. Spironolactone is commenced at 100 mg/day and increased at approximately weekly intervals by 50 mg/day until the maximum tolerated dose of 450 mg/t.d.s. is achieved, or the ascites is controlled and reduced. It is logical to add a small dose of a loop diuretic such as frusemide, 40 mg once or twice a day, to the regimen to enhance sodium and water excretion. It is tempting to speculate whether patients who exfoliate few or no cells into the ascites are more likely to respond to diuretics and aldosterone antagonists than patients shedding numerous cells, but there are no data at present to support this view.

4 *Peritoneovenous shunts*

Shunting malignant ascites into the circulation is not a new concept. Pollock (1975) first described the technique using Spitz-Holter valves designed to drain CSF into the circulation, but this never gained widespread acceptance because the valve was so easily blocked.

Interest in the technique was rekindled by the more recent introduction of larger LeVeen and Denver valves (Fig. 27.1) designed originally to drain ascites from cirrhotic patients, who were refractory to medical therapy, into the superior vena

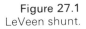

Figure 27.1
LeVeen shunt.

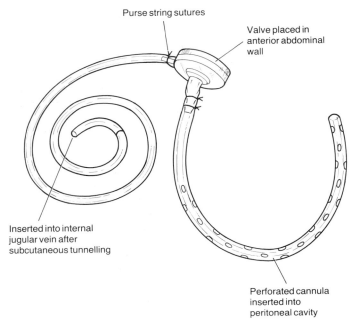

Purse string sutures

Valve placed in
anterior abdominal
wall

Inserted into internal
jugular vein after
subcutaneous tunnelling

Perforated cannula
inserted into
peritoneal cavity

cava. These large valves have achieved considerable success in
this clinical field and the technique has also been applied
successfully in the management of malignant ascites.

Technique
The valves are simple to insert under either a local or,
preferably, a general anaesthesia. The technique is well
described (LeVeen & Wapnick, 1978). The abdominal tube and
the valve chamber are inserted through a small horizontal
right upper quadrant abdominal incision. The tube is tunnelled
subcutaneously and then inserted into the right internal
jugular vein via a small skin crease superclavicular incision. It
is important to drain off a half to three-quarters of the ascites
before inserting the shunt into the vena cava to minimize the
risk of massive and fatal overload. It is also important to
catheterize the patient and administer frusemide, 40 mg intravenously once the valve is in place to encourage a brisk
diuresis and to prevent pulmonary congestion.

The patient requires to be in hospital 2–4 days postoperatively and diuretics, including spironolactone, are continued
postoperatively, not only to delay secretion of ascites but also
to maintain a fairly low central venous pressure. The valves
cease to function and the ascites cease to flow if the venous
pressure equates to the abdominal pressure since a pressure
difference of 3–5 cm H_2O is needed to activate the valves. This
also explains why the valves may not work in the face of

massive ascites which splints the diaphragm, raises intrathoracic pressure, and reduces the normal abdominothoracic pressure differential. Patients should, from time to time, inhale against a resistance to facilitate flow. The simplest way to achieve this is to insert a 5 or 10 ml syringe barrel (without the plunger) into the mouth and inhale through the barrel about five times hourly, exhaling normally. In the case of the Denver valve it is also advisable to pump the chamber five or six times daily to ensure the system is patent and flowing.

Problems

The immediate risk is obviously fluid overload, particularly with tense ascites, but forethought readily avoids this difficulty. Infusing ascitic fluid into the circulation produces a degree of consumptive coagulopathy, possibly because of collagen or thrombin-like protein in the fluid (Ragni et al, 1983). Platelet numbers fall and fibrin degradation products are detectable in blood and urine. However, this process seldom produces clinically important hypocoagulability or bleeding provided the liver is capable of synthesizing clotting factors. Patients at greatest risk of bleeding are those with jaundice and liver failure, an infrequent association with malignant ascites. Longer-term problems are, firstly, the theoretical dissemination of exfoliated malignant cells and widespread metastases formation and, secondly, shunt blockage. There are no reports that shunting malignant ascites into the circulation produces harmful metastases, but there are few detailed studies of the metastasizing potential of peritoneovenous shunts. Tarin et al (1984) observed that about half the patients could develop pulmonary metastases as a consequence of the shunts, but these were of no clinical consequence because of their small size in comparison to the lethal abdominal mass of tumour. The surprising observation is that half the patients appear incapable of developing haematogenous metastases in spite of a continuous infusion of viable, clonogenic malignant cells. Tumour may occasionally implant in the track of the peritoneovenous shunt.

Pulmonary hypertension may, rarely, occur as a result of repeated tumour embolization producing progressive pulmonary capillary block and fibrosis. Thrombus may also form on the venous end of the shunt and in turn embolize. These emboli seldom cause a clinical problem but repeated embolization may contribute to pulmonary hypertension. The most important clinical complication of the shunt is occlusion. This occurs more frequently with malignant ascites than with cirrhotic ascites and is particularly prone to occur in patients with viscid fluid or with ascites with a high fibrin or blood content. Tumour emboli may also occlude the valve. Reaccumulation of the ascites usually signifies shunt occlusion which can be treated, in the case of the Denver valve, by pumping the chamber. It is most commonly the venous end which becomes occluded by a small fibrin plug. Shunt occlusion can be confirmed either by Doppler ultrasound, measurement over the tubing, injection of radioisotope into the peritoneum and scanning over the shunt, or more easily by performing a shuntogram. The needle (21-gauge) of a 20 ml syringe containing about 10 ml of intravenous radio-contrast material, is inserted obliquely through the skin into the efferent tubing under full asepsis. With the needle in the tubing, gentle aspiration of the syringe should withdraw ascites, provided the proximal end of the valve is patent. Injection of the contrast under fluoroscopy will demonstrate the venous end, and the position of the tubing tip. Resistance indicates a fibrin plug which can be safely dislodged by increasing the pressure. Free flow confirms patentcy and care is necessary to prevent cardiac failure due to a subsequent rapid infusion of ascites. Occasionally, flow ceases because venous pressure rises and the shuntogram will confirm patency and allow more appropriate diuretic therapy.

Ultimately, the venous end may become ensheathed in fibrin and cease to function, when a further valve can be inserted, if clinically indicated, either in the other side or via the saphenous vein.

Since shunt insertion requires an operation and a few days in hospital, the selection of the patient for the procedure is important. The main indications are that life expectancy should be at least three months, troublesome ascites reforms rapidly after paracentesis and is refractory to diuretic therapy and appropriate chemotherapy. Used selectively and with close attention to detail postoperatively, the shunts can provide rewarding and useful palliation. However, they are not the first line of treatment.

There are no convincing data at present to determine which of the two peritoneovenous shunts works better in patients with malignant ascites.

Further reading

Anderson, A.T. (1968) Intercavity thiotepa in malignant pleural and peritoneal effusions. *Acta. Radiol. Thor. Phys. Biol.*, 7, 369–378.

Greenway, B., Johnson, P.J. & Williams, R. (1982) Control of malignant ascites with spironolactone. *Br. J. Surg.*, *69*, 441–442.

Henderson, J.M., Stern, S.F., Kutner, M. et al (1980) Analysis of twenty-three plasma protein in ascites. The depletion of fibrinogen and plasminogen. *Ann. Surg.*, *192*, 738–742.

LeVeen, H.H. & Wapnick, S. (1978) Peritoneovenous shunt for ascites. *Surg. Ann.*, *10*, 191–214.

Mitchell, K. & Powell, L.W. (1980) Management of the patient with ascites. *Drugs*, *19*, 383–387.

Paladine, W., Cunningham, T.J. & Sponzo, R. et al (1976) Intracavity bleomycin in the management of malignant effusions. *Cancer*, *38*, 1903–1908.

Pollock, A.V. (1975) The treatment of resistant malignant ascites by insertion of a peritoneo-atrial Holter valve. *Br. J. Surg.*, *62*, 104–107.

Ragni, M.R., Lewis, J.H. & Spero, J.A. (1983) Ascites-induced LeVeen shunt coagulopathy. *Ann. Surg.*, *198*, 91–95.

Slaws, A.K., Roseman, D.L. & Shapiro, T.M. (1979) Peritoneo-venous shunting in the management of malignant ascites. *Arch. Surg.*, *114*, 489–491.

Souter, R.G., Tarin, D. & Kettlewell, M.G.W. (1983) Peritoneo-venous shunts in the management of malignant ascites. *Br. J. Surg.*, *70*, 478–481.

Tarin, D., Price, J.E. & Kettlewell, M.G.W. (1984) Clinical pathological observations on metastasis in man studied in patients treated with peritoneo venous shunts. *Br. Med. J.*, *288*, 749–751.

Tarin, D., Vass, A.C.R., Kettlewell, M.G.W. & Price, J.E. (1984) Absence of metastatic sequelae during long-term treatment of malignant ascites by peritoneo-venous shunting: a clinico-pathological report. *Invasion Metastasis*, *4*, 1–12.

Trotter, J.M., Stueart, J.F.B., McBeth, F. et al (1979) Management of malignant effusion with bleomycin. *Br. J. Cancer*, *40*, 310.

28 Nutritional Complications

Clive Griffith

In patients with cancer, the developing tumour is known to have a profound effect on the nutritional status and metabolism of the host, which may be disproportionate to the size and spread of the tumour, such that the patient's weight frequently falls to one-half of their ideal weight for the last few months of life.

Attempts to reverse the cachectic state seen in patients with disseminated malignant disease, and perhaps improve the response of the tumour to cytotoxic drugs by using aggressive nutritional support, have conferred no clear benefit.

Epidemiological studies have shown that the nutritional status, at the time of diagnosis of patients with cancer, is related to the length of survival after diagnosis and treatment.

Statistical analysis of insurance-policy holders has shown obesity to be related to increased mortality from a variety of cancers. The rates of incidence of colorectal cancer and cancers of breast, endometrium and prostate, may reflect the average annual intake of dietary fat and there is experimental evidence that high-fat diets enhance the growth of murine tumours.

Alternatively, marginal undernutrition in cancer patients (15% and below ideal body weight) is associated with improved survival and dietary calorie restriction is linked with the decreased incidence of some tumours. In the experimental situation, low-protein diets and severe calorie restriction inhibit the growth of implanted tumours in animals, but the sensitivity of the tumour to chemotherapy is reduced.

The nutritional status of cancer patients

The cachectic state associated with cancer is characterized by the syndrome of weight loss, early satiety, anorexia and anaemia. The effects on the nutritional status of the host are clinically evident in the loss of subcutaneous fat and skeletal muscle bulk. Studies of body composition in cancer patients show that fat is lost early but that lean body mass is relatively well preserved until the late stages of the disease. Cancer patients have a generalized increase in total body water but the distribution between the intra- and extracellular compartments remains normal. Total body potassium is reduced, indicating loss of lean-body mass, and hypoalbuminaemia is a feature which, with reduced levels of many enzyme systems, indicates a failure of visceral protein synthesis.

Table 28.1
Factors affecting the
desire to eat.

Altered taste sensation
Altered sense of smell
Nausea
Vomiting
Pain
Satiety
Psychological status
Awareness of underlying disease

Changes in metabolism and nutrition of cancer patients

The cells of a malignant tumour are programmed exclusively for growth and replication, which ultimately results in the death of the tumour-bearing host. The alteration in the host's metabolism in response to the tumour results in the cancer cachexia syndrome which may be seen as a last desperate attempt by the host to limit the intake of calories and protein so as to starve the tumour of energy and nutrients.

The aetiology of cancer cachexia is unknown but many factors are implicated in its causation. The basic defect is an imbalance between the intake of nutrients and energy expenditure by the host. Basal metabolic rate (BMR) is frequently elevated in cancer patients and while subjects without cancer, who are starved, lower their BMR to conserve energy, it tends to remain elevated in starving cancer patients despite calorie restriction.

The mechanisms which control normal food intake are complex and subject to a variety of internal factors which modulate the desire to eat (Table 28.1). Decreased appetite and alterations in taste and smell contribute largely to the reduced intake of nutrients which play a large part in the development of the cachectic state. Cancer patients have an elevated taste threshold for sweetness, but a lowered threshold for bitterness. Psychological depression, in reaction to the awareness of advancing malignancy, is a further important factor to the anorexia; however, there may be changes at a hypothalamic level, possibly mediated by tumour metabolites that alter the desire to eat.

The central control of appetite involves serotonin as a neuro-transmitter, and increased central turnover is associated with decreased food intake. Experiments with tumour-bearing rats have shown that tryptophan, an essential amino acid for all animal species including man, is increased in tumour-bearing rats prior to the onset of anorexia. Raised central tryptophan levels result in increased serotonin turnover, which is found in high concentrations in areas of the brain concerned with food intake in anorectic rats. Recent trials of a serotonin antagonist (BC 105) in cancer patients without gastrointestinal tract obstruction, whose cachexia was secondary to widespread malignancy, have been encouraging: there was an increased food intake and body weight with an associated reduction in depressive symptoms.

Protein metabolism in advanced malignancy

Protein stores are depleted in the advanced cancer patient with loss of skeletal muscle bulk and hypoalbuminaemia. Attempts have been made to parallel the clinical similarity between the malnutrition seen following starvation in non-malignant subjects with the cachectic state seen in cancer. Fasting patients with cancer, however, have up to 35% elevation of whole body protein turnover compared to benign starving patients and, similarly, protein synthesis, measured by radioisotope techniques, is up to 50% higher in cancer patients. This demonstrates that, unlike the benign patient who adapts to starvation by reducing protein synthesis and turnover, the patient with cancer when deprived of exogenous calories and nitrogen may continue to have raised protein turnover rates. The protein synthesis rate of the malignant tumour does not, however, appear to be increased over the tissue of origin of the tumour, which suggests that tumour-directed changes of host metabolism by tumour products (such as novel peptides or growth factors) are responsible for the elevation of protein turnover. Novel peptides have been isolated in the urine of patients with malignant disease,

Figure 28.1
The tumour as a
nitrogen 'trap'.

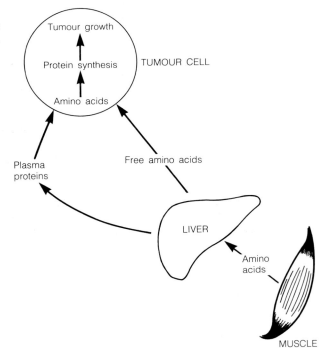

particularly leukaemia, which may be responsible in some part for the chaotic metabolism of these patients.

Even when adequate amino acids and calories are supplied to the tumour-bearing patient, net losses of nitrogen occur with loss to the tumour which may act as a nitrogen trap (Fig. 28.1). Cancer patients also show abnormal amino acid profiles, indicating continuing gluconeogenesis from amino acids derived from host-protein stores to supply the energy requirements of the tumour.

Fat metabolism

There is a clinically-obvious loss of total body fat in the patient with progressive malignancy, although phospholipid and free cholesterol content may increase. Lipid is mobilized to excess in the cancer patient to provide energy for oxidative metabolism. High serum levels of free fatty acids are found with increased rates of clearance leading to progressive depletion of endogenous fat stores. This phenomenon occurs at an early stage in the development of the tumour, which may be due to either a tumour-directed increase in plasma lipase activity or the production of lipolytic factors by the tumour. Exogenous fat, as, for example, part of an intravenous feeding regimen, is also rapidly cleared from the circulation.

Glucose metabolism

Patients with cancer tend to have a diabetic type of glucose tolerance, due to both the production of abnormal insulins and peripheral insulin resistance. Increased gluconeogenesis from amino acids, broken down from skeletal and visceral protein stores, may also contribute to the hyperglycaemia.

In patients with metastatic breast cancer, the secretory capacity of the pancreas to produce insulin is reduced and this becomes even lower following hypophysectomy when the stimulatory effect of growth hormone on the pancreatic B cells is removed.

Tumour cell metabolism is characterized by anaerobic glucose metabolism with the generation of lactic acid as the end-product, which is recycled via the Cori cycle (Fig. 28.2) activity of the liver and kidney. This is a very inefficient process in terms of energy expenditure with a net loss of high energy phosphate, when compared to the aerobic conversion of one mole of lactic acid to glucose by the Krebs cycle, which generates 30 moles of ATP. The increased activity of the Cori cycle in the cancer patient

Figure 28.2
The Cori cycle.

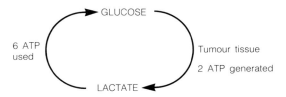

6 ATP used

GLUCOSE

Tumour tissue

2 ATP generated

LACTATE

represents a considerable energy drain which is responsible in some part for the cancer cachexia syndrome.

All body tissues and organs in the cancer patient lose weight except the liver, which gains weight due to an increase in both total water content and dry weight. The reason for this phenomenon remains unknown.

Nutritional support in the cancer patient

With the advent of nutritional support techniques, particularly total parenteral nutrition (TPN), it was hoped that the nutritional depletion of the patient with advanced cancer and the wide-ranging metabolism derangement caused by the tumour could be reversed.

Malnutrition in cancer patients, including those with breast cancer, is associated with reduced response rates to chemotherapy. The growth rate of the tumour may decrease as the weight of the host falls, allowing tumour cells to enter a non-proliferative phase rendering them less sensitive to growth-specific chemotherapeutic agents, and conversely, nutritional support of the host could alter tumour growth kinetics to favour lysis by such agents.

Nutritional support in the form of total parenteral nutrition has been of proven benefit in patients with gastrointestinal tract cancer undergoing resectional surgery, with reduction of wound infection, intra-abdominal and pulmonary sepsis, and anastomotic leakage in the postoperative period. The anxiety that aggressive nutritional support might enhance the growth rate of the tumour has been largely dispelled by Mullen and his colleagues who showed that protein-synthesis rates of tumours in patients receiving intravenous feeding were no greater than from the surrounding tissues from which the tumours arose.

The reversal or amelioration of the cachexia in patients with advanced tumours by using supplementary nutrition (particularly TPN) could be seen as a possible way to improve response rates to chemotherapy. Many chemotherapeutic drugs produce nausea and vomiting which compounds the anorexia of the patient with advanced cancer and makes the use of intravenous nutritional support an attractive possibility.

Initial non-randomized trials of intravenous nutritional support with chemotherapy for solid tumours (including breast carcinomas) gave encouraging results in terms of improved well-being, reduction of gastrointestinal toxicity, and reversal of weight loss, but offered no dramatic improvement of response to chemotherapy.

The first randomized controlled clinical trial of TPN as an adjunct to chemotherapy was conducted in patients with metastatic colorectal cancer, who showed improved weight gain but minimal changes in anthropometric measures, such as arm muscle circumference, and a decrease in serum albumin, when compared to the control group receiving chemotherapy alone.

This study also showed that chemotherapy plus parenteral nutrition did not confer a survival advantage over the non-fed groups.

Other trials of TPN plus chemotherapy in anaplastic small-cell lung cancer showed no benefit in terms of general health, reduction of side-effects such as nausea and vomiting, or improvement in response rates to chemotherapy; similarly, TPN is known to be ineffective in preventing chemotherapy-induced myelosuppression.

A small uncontrolled study of Adriamycin plus TPN in Japanese women with breast cancer refractory to other treatment, was reported as encouraging, showing an improved tolerance to chemotherapy and some evidence of a clinical response.

The overall impression, however, of the use of total parenteral nutrition as an adjunct to cancer chemotherapy is that response rates are not improved and survival is not prolonged. Although body weight is preserved in the patients receiving supplementary intravenous feeding, lean body mass is not improved and TPN is ineffective in reversing the metabolic and nutritional effects of the tumour in patients with advanced cancer.

Nutritional support for the patient with advanced breast cancer

The diet for the patient with advanced cancer should take account of her depressed mental state and abnormalities of taste and should be attractively presented. Various high-calorie and high-protein liquid feeds can be made by the hospital dieticians or supplied directly by drug companies, which are sometimes useful in providing supplementary nutrition for the cancer patient.

Nutritional support, particularly intravenous nutrition in the advanced cancer patient, is a contentious subject since it is now well recognized that nutritional therapy fails to reverse the metabolic effects on the host; however, it may in selected patients improve the sense of well-being and help them to cope with the side-effects of prolonged chemotherapy, such as nausea and vomiting.

In breast cancer patients with direct involvement of the gastrointestinal tract due to omental, peritoneal or nodal metastases, and who are clinically nutritionally depleted, there may be a role for supplementary intravenous nutrition if a gastrointestinal anastomosis from resection or bypass of the lesion requires to be fashioned. Similarly, patients with advanced breast cancer who require extensive plastic procedures such as a latissimus dorsi flap to cover skin defects following mastectomy, may benefit from nutritional support in the pre- and perioperative period for two to three weeks before returning to full oral diet.

The principles of intravenous nutrition are now well established. All solutions should be given through a central venous silastic catheter inserted via the internal jugular or subclavian

Figure 28.3
A patient having
intravenous nutrition
given by subclavian
line.

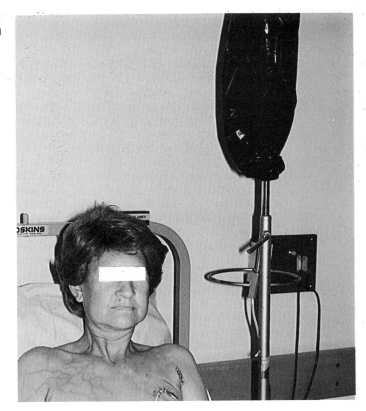

venous route (Fig. 28.3). An alternative is a cut down onto the
cephalic vein with advancement into the subclavian. A skin
tunnel of 4–6 inches is essential between the skin entry site of the
catheter and the site of venous entry. Rigorous attention to
aseptic technique during insertion and subsequent care of the
catheter is essential; lines from the catheter to the feeding
solution should be changed daily. A simple regime should be
followed—10–15 g of nitrogen in the form of a proprietary amino
acid solution with 2000–2500 calories, one-third supplied by fat
(intralipid) with the remaining two-thirds as dextrose. For those
hospitals fortunate enough to have a laminar air flow facility in
the pharmacy, the total feeding solution, including fat and
essential water and fat-soluble vitamins plus trace elements, can
be made up in a 3 litre bag to be infused over 12–24 hours,
otherwise intravenous feeding can be achieved using multiple
bottles of amino acid and calories (fat and dextrose) providing
both are infused simultaneously.

Complications of total parenteral nutrition
The complications of total parenteral nutrition can be divided

into those related to the central venous catheter and those related to the feeding solution used.

Catheter-related complications

Sepsis is the main problem; because of the direct access to the central veins it can rapidly produce a fatal septicaemia. Scrupulous aspesis in placing the catheter, ideally in the operating theatre, and a long subcutaneous tunnel separating the skin entry site from the site of venepuncture have reduced septic episodes to under 1%. Catheter care is the responsibility of the nursing staff, or the patient if home treatment is undertaken, and should involve aseptic techniques for change of drip tubing from the feeding solution to the catheter and daily flushing with heparinized saline.

Other problems related to the catheter are air embolism, which can be averted by clamping the catheter when changing the drip tubing, catheter blockage, which should not occur if daily flushing with heparinized saline is carried out, and, finally, catheter dislodgement which usually requires replacement of the catheter.

Complications related to the feeding solution

Hyperosmolar dehydration is caused by giving dextrose faster than it can be metabolized, causing an osmotic diuresis which results in coma and ultimately death. If the energy source used is divided between dextrose and fat, this should not occur and the use of supplementary insulin is usually unnecessary.

Fluid overload can be caused in elderly patients or those with poor cardiac reserve and is prevented by reducing the volume of the solution infused.

Other complications are rare and are only manifest in long-term intravenous feeding and include trace element deficiencies, vitamin deficiencies and also fatty liver replacement.

Tube feeding

If the gastrointestinal tract is functioning and the patient is able to tolerate nutrition by the enteral route, then fine-bore tube feeding is an attractive possibility if the patient's nutritional state is causing concern.

Fine-bore enteral feeding tubes are passed into the stomach, duodenum or in some cases the small bowel if there is evidence of gastric stasis.

Specially formulated liquid diets are prepared aseptically by the hospital dietitian or, alternatively, many liquid diets are commercially available. All are designed with a high protein content with adequate calories, vitamins and electrolytes to support the patient's nutritional requirements. The delivery system is simple with a 1.5 or 2 litre reservoir connected by tubing to the fine-bore feeding tube, using either gravity or a small pump to allow delivery of the feeding solution over the desired time period.

Diarrhoea occurs in up to 20% of patients and can be regulated by either slowing the rate of delivery or alternatively using anti-diarrhoeal agents such as Lomotil or loperamide in the feeding solution.

Many patients initially complain of abdominal distension and bloating but this can be avoided by starting with one-quarter strength feeds, building up to full strength after two or three days.

Oesophageal complications seen with the wider-bore Ryle's tube are fortunately extremely rare with the modern fine-bore silastic tubes.

Future perspectives

Further research into the cachexia associated with advanced malignant disease and improved understanding of the pathophysiology of the syndrome, particularly at the central level, will undoubtedly lead to effective agents to improve the anorexia and depressed mood of these patients and allow them to eat normally.

Although aggressive nutritional support in patients with advanced cancer has failed to improve response to chemotherapy or prolong survival, future therapies with tailored amino acid solutions which benefit the host preferentially may prove more effective. Future studies of the relationship of tumour growth to the supply of specific exogenous nutrients may enable suppression of tumour growth to enhance the effect of specific antitumour agents which inhibit various parts of the cycle of tumour growth.

Although it is inevitable that the patient with advanced and disseminated breast cancer will become grossly undernourished, supplementary nutrition either by the enteral or parenteral route may be indicated where prolonged nausea and vomiting, secondary to powerful chemotherapeutic drugs, have made the patient's life a misery. Despite advancing malignant disease, the patient, who is provided with adequate calories and nitrogen, often benefits from an improved mental attitude and state of well-being, compared to those who are denied such support.

Further reading

Brennan, M.F. & Copeland, E.M. (1981) Panel report on nutritional support of patients with cancer. *Am. J. Clin. Nutr.*, *34*, 1199–1205.

Busby, G.P. & Steinberg, J.J. (1981) Nutrition in cancer patients. *Surg. Clin. N. America*, *61*, 691–700.

DeWys, W.D., Begg, C., Band, P. & Tormey, D. (1981) The impact of malnutrition on treatment results in breast cancer. *Cancer Treatment Reports*, *65(5)*, 87–91.

Theologides, A. (1979) Cancer cachexia. *Cancer*, *43*, 2004–2012.

Tominoga, T., Onodera, T., Kitamura, M. et al (1980) Combined treatment by chemotherapy and intravenous hyperalimentation in Japanese patients with advanced breast cancer. *Cancer*, *46*, 642–646.

Wesdorp, R.I.C., Krause, R.M. & Meyen Feldt, A. (1983) Cancer cachexia and its nutritional implications. *Br. J. Surg.*, *70*, 352–355.

29 Hypercalcaemia

Charles Campbell

All attempts to achieve an improvement of breast cancer mortality have concentrated upon earlier and more effective anticancer therapies and little attention has been paid to the treatment of cancer-related disorders which themselves may cause serious morbidity or death. Hypercalcaemia is a common cancer-related condition which may occur with minimal or undetectable metastases, may progress rapidly, and usually poses a much more immediate threat to life than the cancer itself.

Ten to twenty per cent of all women with breast cancer will develop hypercalcaemia at some time during the evolution of their disease, usually in the presence of clinically detectable bone secondaries. Since the cancer is clearly incurable at this stage, the question arises as to whether active treatment of the calcium disturbance is appropriate. Judgement is required. Treatment of hypercalcaemia is simple and safe and there can be little argument against its use in patients with limited bone metastases. In the absence of hypercalcaemia, these women would be expected to have a fairly long survival (median interval 15–18 months). They may be entirely pain-free or it may be controlled by radiotherapy or a variety of measures provided by the pain specialist. Treatment of hypercalcaemia in these patients, therefore, would provide a worthwhile prolongation of good quality survival. Few clinicians would wish to prolong the suffering of patients who are terminally ill with extensive metastases in lungs, liver or brain as well as bone, and any treatment to lower serum calcium in these patients should be intended for symptomatic relief only.

Pathophysiology

An understanding of the sequence of events leading to hypercalcaemia is essential if treatment is to be effective. In metastatic breast cancer, calcium homeostasis is maintained when the excess which is resorbed by tumour deposits in bone is excreted by the kidney. The normal kidney has a considerable capacity for calcium excretion and the urinary clearance only becomes incomplete when the calcium load is very large. Thus, the majority of women with bone secondaries are normocalcaemic, but they have a high urinary excretion of calcium which is significantly greater than that of patients with soft-tissue metastases.

When the equilibrium between the increased calcium resorption on one hand and increased renal clearance on the other is disturbed, hypercalcaemia will result. Typical events which will disturb this equilibrium include:

1 *Dehydration*
Patients with advanced breast cancer are prone to vomiting, due either to the effect of the tumour itself or to anticancer therapy. Dehydration quickly impairs the urinary excretion of calcium and initiates hypercalcaemia.

2 *Immobilization*
Patients with painful bone secondaries who take to bed increase the site of calcium resorption from bone simply due to immobilization. The increase in calcium load may be sufficient to overwhelm the kidneys' excretory capacity.

3 *Bone destruction*
Rapid bone destruction due to an aggressive tumour may have a sufficiently high calcium load to exceed renal handling and present de novo, with hypercalcaemia.

A further complicating factor is that an elevation of serum calcium itself impairs glomerular and tubular function, thus limiting the homeostatic function of the kidney. Therefore, a vicious circle starts with an event which causes an alteration of the calcium clearance equilibrium which leads to an elevation of serum calcium. Hypercalcaemia itself leads to progressive impairment of renal-tubular concentrating capacity, dehydration, a further fall in renal calcium excretion and a further rise in serum calcium. Thus, hypercalcaemia associated with breast cancer has skeletal and renal components and once established it may progress rapidly. The rate of progress is related to the magnitude of the calcium load presented to the kidney and the degree of disturbance of homeostasis. Patients with mild hypercalcaemia may remain clinically well for many weeks before becoming progressively worse, whereas those with severe hypercalcaemia (3 mmol/litre) at first detection are usually dehydrated, have some degree of uraemia, and the disturbance usually becomes rapidly worse. If left untreated, hypercalcaemia may cause permanent renal damage, making calcium balance unstable and subsequent homeostasis more difficult to attain. Early appropriate therapy can, however, restore renal function to normal and early recognition of the disorder would be clearly advantageous.

Clinical features
Patients who remain normocalcaemic despite a high rate of bone resorption and a high urinary excretion of calcium may be wholly asymptomatic or may complain of mild urinary frequency. Mild hypercalcaemia may be similarly symptom-free and, unfortunately, clinical features are scant or absent until the disorder is at a

relatively advanced state. Thus, clinical detection of the disorder at an early stage is difficult.

Symptoms associated with severe hypercalcaemia (3 mmol/ litre) are troublesome and include weakness, fatigue, drowsiness, depression, nausea, vomiting and constipation. On examination, patients may be found to be dehydrated with a tachycardia. Muscular hypotonia is quite common.

Detection of calcium disturbances in breast cancer

The main difficulty associated with developing or established hypercalcaemia of breast cancer is its detection. Onset of clinical symptoms may be rapid and the patient may be admitted apparently close to death, semicomatose and vomiting.

Clearly, clinical recognition is unreliable due to an absence of features associated with the early disorder and because of the rather non-specific symptoms and signs associated with the advanced stage. The vigilant clinician may recognize hypercalcaemia in a hospitalized patient, but the majority of women with metastatic breast cancer are managed as out-patients and are at relatively high risk of hypercalcaemia, particularly if they are prone to vomiting or if they take to bed for any length of time. Sudden, unexpected deaths at home of stable women with bone secondaries are not uncommon and it is possible that many of these have been due to hypercalcaemia.

Regular measurements of serum calcium at the out-patient clinic are easy to perform, but they tell us nothing about the early stages of calcium disturbance. As outlined previously, serum calcium only becomes elevated when homeostasis is lost, and once raised it can progress very rapidly. Thus, it is possible for a woman to be seen at an out-patient clinic with a normal serum calcium one week and to be admitted as an emergency with severe hypercalcaemia the next.

Urinary calcium is a much more sensitive indicator of the early alterations of homeostasis than serum values, but the conventional 24 hour measurement is tedious and collections are frequently inaccurate.

To get around this difficulty, Nordin introduced the test of Ca_E (calcium excretion per litre glomerular filtrate) which is simply a urinary calcium measurement corrected for the creatinine clearance and is calculated by the equation:

$$Ca_E = \frac{\text{Urinary calcium excretion}}{\text{Creatinine clearance}}$$

$$= \frac{\text{Urinary calcium} \times \dfrac{\text{Volume}}{\text{Time}}}{\dfrac{\text{Urinary creatinine}}{\text{Serum creatinine}}}$$

$$= \frac{\text{Urine calcium}}{\text{Urine creatinine}} \times \text{Serum creatinine mmol/l}$$

Urine volume and collection time cancel in both numerator and denominator which obviates the need for timed urine volumes and the test can be performed upon 'spot' samples of blood and urine.

This test is simplicity itself and is ideal in that it takes account of changes of renal function which, as outlined previously, is important in the maintenance of calcium homeostasis. In practice, patients are asked to bring a fasting 20 ml sample of urine to the clinic, which is sent for calcium and creatinine assays. At the clinic a 10 ml sample of blood is taken for estimation of albumin, calcium and creatinine. Serum calcium measurements are corrected to a reference serum albumin of 40 g/litre using the formula.

Corrected serum calcium
= measured serum calcium
+ 0.02 (40 − serum albumin)

Once corrected, the simple calculation for Ca_E can be carried out. This test gives a good estimate of calcium resorption from bone. Most patients with bone secondaries have values in excess of 30 mmol/litre glomerular filtrate, although values may fall with a response to systemic therapy or rise with disease progression or relapse. Our data suggests that patients with rising values of Ca_E are at high risk of hypercalcaemia.

This test, in summary, is ideal for monitoring calcium balance at the out-patient clinic and ought to be carried out in all patients with an early recurrence at any site or who are judged to be at risk of early recurrence on the basis of large tumour size and lymph-node involvement at mastectomy.

Treatment of established hypercalcaemia
As outlined, hypercalcaemia has skeletal and renal components. The initial abnormality is a raised calcium load from bone resorption which, by the mechanism outlined, leads to loss of renal-tubular concentrating capacity, dehydration and worsening of the hypercalcaemia. Consequently, treatment ought to be given in the reverse order, with volume depletion being corrected first before the suppression of the resorption.

Correction of dehydration   Salt and water replacement is a simple and highly effective remedy for reducing the serum calcium. Normal saline is preferable in this context to any other volume expander since calcium reabsorption in the nephron is linked to that of sodium. Consequently, provision of sodium excess by saline infusion promotes sodium excretion as well as that of calcium.

Treatment is begun after single-venous blood and untimed urine samples have been obtained for Ca_E. One-half to one litre of 0.9% saline is given every 6 hours for 48 hours. During this time, the patient's condition can be made more comfortable by the use of anti-emetic for nausea and other symptomatic agents. Rehydration may be judged to be complete when urinary output is satisfactory and blood urea levels lie within the normal range, and it is virtually always achieved within 48 hours.

Correction of the renal component of hypercalcaemia in this manner may restore serum calcium to normal levels, or it may remain slightly elevated, and this is accompanied by a clinical improvement of circulatory, cerebral and renal function. If treatment were to be discontinued at this point, then relapse would be likely since the high rate of calcium resorption from bone which initiated the loss of homeostasis, would remain uncontrolled.

Suppression of calcium resorption After rehydration has been completed, serum calcium often falls to within the normal range, but Ca_E values usually remain high due to bone resorption. Thus a further Ca_E measurement taken at the end of rehydration provides a very good measurement of calcium resorption and is a good guide of the effectiveness of the second line of treatment.

Suppression of calcium resorption should be carried out initially with the least toxic agents, and salmon calcitonin in a dose of 100 IU three times daily is effective in many patients. Treatment should be continued in this dosage for one week and then be reduced to a maintenance dose of 100 IU which may be administered by the patient herself subcutaneously. Treatment can be continued over long intervals and anaphylactic reactions are rare. Mithramycin is a particularly effective agent which should be used in patients who are resistant to salmon calcitonin. This drug is a cytotoxic antibiotic, which when used in high doses as an anti-cancer agent, is toxic and causes bone marrow suppression and impairment of renal function. Much smaller doses are used to achieve suppression of calcium resorption in the treatment of hypercalcaemia and side-effects are few. Corticosteroids are ineffective in achieving a suppression of bone resorption and have little part to play in the management of hypercalcaemia due to breast cancer.

Long-term maintenance
Maintenance of calcium homeostasis is dependent upon a number of factors, including the degree of renal damage produced by the hypercalcaemia, the duration of suppression of calcium resorption by specific therapy, and the presence or absence of a response to systemic anti-cancer therapy. Clearly, women who achieve a response to systemic endocrine or cytotoxic chemotherapy would be likely to achieve good long-term calcium homeostasis. Monitoring of patients may be carried out by serial estimations of Ca_E as well as of serum calcium at outpatient clinics, and a repetition of treatment is indicated when either of these show a rapid rate of rise.

Prevention of hypercalcaemia
Prevention of hypercalcaemia would avoid the complications of

permanent renal damage and it is clearly preferable to treatment of established diseases. Logically, all patients with metastases who have a high Ca_E would be expected to obtain long-lasting benefit from treatment effecting a reduction of calcium resorption. However, the agents (calcitonin, mithramycin) are very expensive and treatment is rather inconvenient for patients. Before a statutory recommendation for this treatment in asymptomatic women can be issued further clinical studies are necessary to demonstrate:

- the effectiveness of Ca_E in selecting patients most at risk;
- the effectiveness of calcitonin or mithramycin in preventing hypercalcaemia.
- a worthwhile survival benefit.

Further reading

Benabe, J.E. & Martinez Maldonado, M. (1978) Hypercalcaemic nephropathy. *Arch. Intern. Med.*, *138*, 777–779.

Campbell, F.C., Blamey, R.W., Woolfson, A.M.J., Elston, C.W. & Hosking, D.J. (1983) Calcium excretion (Ca_E) in metastatic breast cancer. *Br. J. Surg.*, *70*, 202–204.

Hosking, D.J., Cowley, A. & Bucknall, C.A. (1981) Rehydration in the treatment of severe hypercalcaemia. *Q. J. Med.*, *50*, 473–481.

Lins, L.E. (1979) Renal function in hypercalcaemia. *Acta. Med. Scand. (Suppl).*, *206*, 8–46.

Nordin, B.E. & Peacock, M. (1969) Role of the kidney in regulation of plasma calcium. *Lancet*, *12*, 1280–1283.

30 Psychological Complications of Advanced Breast Cancer

Penelope Hopwood

Although there has now been extensive research into the psychosocial sequelae of early breast cancer and its treatment, comparatively little attention has been focused on the plight of patients with progressive disease. Such patients may have to face increasing loss of body integrity and function, pain from disease, treatment toxicity and the difficulty of coming to terms with a fatal condition. The psychological impact of these problems may be considerable, and a proportion of women will develop psychiatric morbidity. Such morbidity, its recognition and treatment will be discussed.

Psychiatric morbidity

It is all too often assumed that breaking bad news to patients will inevitably result in some kind of catastrophic reaction. Fears of precipitating feelings of hopelessness and even suicide have often prevented clinicians from disclosing that the disease is progressing.

However, in recent years there has been a trend towards more openness with patients and a greater preparedness to discuss the disease and its treatment. A major factor in these changes has been the use of chemotherapy, for this has necessitated revealing disease status in order to justify the use of medication which may cause considerable toxicity. As clinicians more frequently practise an open approach, it is apparent that most patients cope well, and only a minority find it difficult to adjust. There are no general rules about what to tell or not to tell patients with progressive disease. Instead, information must be tailored to the individual and what she indicates she wants or does not want to know. An approach which is sensitive to her cues, allows the patient to enquire if she wants to, but maintains hope, will often prevent a morbid reaction occurring.

Those who still experience difficulty coping with advanced cancer are likely to develop a depressive illness or anxiety state.

Depressive illness

Clinically significant depression has been found to occur in 20–30% of a heterogeneous group of cancer patients admitted for the treatment of advanced disease (Plumb and Holland, 1981). This level of morbidity was confirmed in our study of 26 women suffering from advanced breast cancer, of whom 9 had an affective disorder. Depressive illness predominated although anxiety symptoms were usually also present. Anxiety states alone were much less common (4%). Depression is clearly reactive in the majority of patients and due to the discovery of progressive disease or adverse effects of treatment. It has often been said that because such depression is 'understandable' it is therefore not worth treating. This view has hindered the detection and treatment of depressive disorder. However, a patient will usually recognize that her distress represents a distinct departure from normal and report that she cannot 'shake off' her low mood and that her fears have persisted for several weeks. These are characteristic features of depressive illness.

The symptoms of depressive illness are described in Chapter 15. Clearly, it can be more difficult to ascribe some symptoms (like anergia, loss of weight, anorexia) to a depressive illness in a woman with advanced disease, since they may also be attributable to the growth of her cancer. A full evaluation of both physical and psychological status is required. Anhedonic features (such as failing to take pleasure in activities, loss of interest in appearance), together with feelings of guilt or hopelessness, tearfulness and irritability, may also indicate depressive illness. In advanced cancer, the patient's functional capacity may already have been compromised, and depression may significantly aggravate this. She will find it hard to distract herself from worries because of poor concentration and loss of interest; thus, the quality of life can be substantially reduced. Furthermore, her ability to tolerate pain and other symptoms like breathlessness may be considerably reduced when depression coexists. In contrast to early breast cancer, advanced disease is quite frequently associated with pain caused by metastatic disease. The presence of depression is known to adversely affect the control of such pain.

Depression may also reduce the patient's tolerance to adverse effects of treatment, especially the toxicity of chemotherapy or radiotherapy. Then, if mood disorder is severe, the patient may refuse further treatment.

Anxiety states

Up to one-quarter of women presenting with advanced disease may report anxiety symptoms, although a frank anxiety state in the absence of depressive illness is much less common. An anxiety state is a pathological level of anxiety which is out of character for the patient, affects her normal function, and does not remit spontaneously. It is characterized by preoccupying worries, irritability, poor concentration, a feeling of nervousness or by marked somatic symptoms such as palpitations, breathlessness, sweating, tremor and faintness. Such symptoms may be wrongly attributed by the patient to the effects of cancer, and so cause further anxiety, thus establishing a vicious circle. Clearly, a degree of anxiety is appropriate to the discovery of disease progression. For example, a patient may feel 'worried sick' for a few days after hearing bad news, lose some sleep because of this, and be unable to concentrate on reading the newspaper. However, she is soon able to distract herself from her worries, her sleep pattern reverts to normal, she responds to reassurance and feels she is 'coming to terms' with the new problem she faces. This transient reaction which results in adjustment, must be distinguished from a morbid reaction through relevant enquiry.

As in the postmastectomy situation, anxiety states may be complicated by an irrational fear (phobia) of specific situations such as going out of the house. This condition, agoraphobia, may further compromise the patient's functional level and hence quality of life. Phobic anxiety, as opposed to generalized anxiety, may also develop in relation to treatments such as radiotherapy, and in particular, chemotherapy.

The psychological effect of chemotherapy

Although psychological problems develop in patients not receiving active treatment, or in those receiving hormone therapy or radiotherapy, certain specific difficulties are associated with chemotherapy and warrant separate mention. The problem of treatment-related nausea and vomiting is becoming a growing concern to many clinicians, particularly as these symptoms are often unrelieved by conventional antiemetics (Chapter 22). A psychological component has been suggested, especially to the nausea and vomiting that occurs in anticipation of chemotherapy. Vomiting may occur reflexly prior to chemotherapy and this mechanism is now attributed to Pavlovian conditioning aggravated by anxiety (Nesse et al, 1980). This may be either general anxiety, with nausea and vomiting occurring in response to vague stimuli, or is associated with the specific taste, sight or smell of chemotherapy. In one study (Altmaier et al, 1982) vomiters were found to be significantly more depressed, as well as more anxious, than non-vomiters, suggesting that the patients' perceived lack of control and negative thoughts may be contributory. Although 'conditioned' vomiting more frequently complicates potential treatment, it can also occur with oral chemotherapy. The patient's sense of failure in being unable to control her symptoms, aggravates her psychological problems.

Alopecia may also provoke or contribute to psychiatric morbidity, as was described for the adjuvant chemotherapy situation. The blow to a woman's loss of femininity may seem even harder to bear, however, when treatment is known to be palliative. Further, losing her hair may rekindle earlier distressing feelings about the loss of the breast, and thereby aggravate depressive or anxiety symptoms.

*Organic
brain syndrome*
Confusional states may complicate advanced breast cancer and its treatment and result in disturbed behaviour which makes management difficult. Such states are characterized by an altered level of consciousness, disorientation (in time, place, person), impaired cognitive function, and agitation. A more frank disturbance in which visual hallucinations and disordered thought occurs can mimic a psychotic illness.

The speed of onset and course will tend to reflect the underlying organic cause and this may include hypercalcaemia, cerebral metastases or severe infection complicating cytotoxic treatment.

Recognition of psychiatric morbidity
Although it has been demonstrated in research studies that psychiatric morbidity associated with breast cancer and its treatment can be identified and evaluated, such problems may frequently go unrecognized in routine clinical practice. This phenomenon of 'hidden morbidity' is intricately associated with a more general issue concerning doctor–patient communication in oncology (Chapter 15). Although some research studies have referred to the problem of recognition, few have addressed it specifically. Furthermore, when psychiatric morbidity presents in an atypical fashion, it is acknowledged that its identification may be even more difficult. For instance, the agitation of a depressive illness may be misdiagnosed as overactivity and the patient labelled as 'disturbed' or 'difficult'. Lack of motivation or excessive dependence on ward staff may be misinterpreted as poor patient compliance, but, again, it may mask depression. Up to a quarter of patients referred for psychiatric assessment may be misclassified by the referring doctor (Hinton, 1972). The area of cognitive function is also likely to be overlooked or misinterpreted, and is frequently unreported. It has been found that patients who are disturbed or uncooperative are more likely to be referred for psychiatric assessment, and in such patients organic brain syndrome may be a frequent diagnosis (Levine et al, 1978). Up to two-thirds of these patients may be misdiagnosed by the referring physician. Any change in cognitive function in patients with advanced disease should first be investigated on a physical basis to exclude cerebral metastases, hypercalcaemia or other metabolic upset, before assuming a psychological basis.

The non-disclosure of side-effects in patients receiving chemotherapy, or sometimes even hormone therapy, may also provide difficulties in clinical practice. Patients fear being labelled 'ungrateful' if they complain about treatment, or worry lest their treatment be discontinued. Clinicians may therefore be misled as to how therapy is being tolerated, which may result in inappropriate management or poor compliance. If conditioned vomiting develops, patients often do not report their difficulties until they are on the point of opting out of further treatment.

Improving recognition In order to achieve the best possible quality of life for patients with advanced breast cancer, it is essential to try and evaluate a woman's psychological adjustment and, where indicated, offer help. It behoves the surgeon to ask open questions and to be alert to patients' cues in order to recognize psychological morbidity.

1 *Open questions*

This approach has been described in Chapter 15. The surgeon can acknowledge that psychological problems may develop during the treatment of advanced cancer and facilitate their disclosure. For instance, he may say that: 'We know that some ladies get depressed in this situation; how have you been feeling?' or 'Some ladies become very upset when they start to lose their hair; how is it affecting you?' General questions of this sort quickly help to establish whether or not such problems exist.

2 *Responding to cues*

In the advanced disease situation the patient's cues may easily be missed when attention is focused on her physical status. For instance, if a patient comments: 'I've not been feeling so good, doctor', it is tempting to follow this with an enquiry such as: 'Oh, has your pain been worse?' The woman may then feel that it is inappropriate to disclose her emotions. Rather, the surgeon should respond with: 'In what way have you not been feeling well? Do you mean something physical?' or 'How have you been feeling in general about the way things are?'

In a similar way, clues to treatment toxicity, conditioned vomiting or anxiety symptoms can be followed up, rather than dismissed with statements of false reassurance such as 'I'm sure you'll be all right next time'.

Clinicians frequently comment that using open questions and responding to patients' cues may lead to a time-consuming conversation. An alternative strategy is to acknowledge to the patient that her problem has been noticed and arrange to put more time aside on another occasion to deal with it. This can give the patient some relief, and facilitate more direct disclosure at the subsequent visit.

3 *Screening*

It has been found that patients will report psychological symptoms using some kind of self-report questionnaire even though they fail to complain spontaneously of being distressed (Farber et al, 1982). We have used this approach successfully in patients with advanced breast cancer. Ideally, such questionnaires should be short, so as not to overtax ill patients, should be acceptable to patients, to ensure compliance, and should be easy to administer by staff without psychiatric training. A wide variety of questionnaires has now been constructed for use in hospital settings, although many lack clinical validity (that is, the ability to discriminate accurately patients who are psychologically well or ill). Some, such as the Hospital Anxiety and Depression Scale (Zigmond and Snaith, 1983), the General Health Questionnaire (Goldberg, 1972), and the Rotterdam Symptom Checklist (de Haes et al, 1983) appear to have potential but require specific validation in advanced breast cancer patients. A linear analogue self-assessment scale (LASA) has proved useful in comparing the effects of different treatment regimes in breast cancer patients (Baum et al, 1980), but it does not fulfil the role of a screening instrument for individual patients.

4 *Specialist nurses*
The value of specialist nurses working with patients after mastectomy has been reported (Chapter 15), and some of these patients had already developed progressive disease. However, no systemic evaluation of this role has been carried out in women with advanced breast cancer.

Treatment of psychiatric morbidity
Using the techniques and resources outlined above, the surgeon can quickly become aware of psychological problems in his patients and decide on appropriate management. When psychological disorder is severe or complex, the patient may need to be referred for more detailed psychiatric assessment. With other patients the surgeon may wish to alert the general practitioner to the problem, or prescribe medication in the out-patient clinic.

Depressive illness

1 *Antidepressant medication*
Antidepressive medication should be used when depressive illness develops in a patient with advanced disease. Even when it cannot be foreseen that a complete 6 month course can be completed it is important to try and relieve depressive symptoms promptly and maintain treatment as long as possible. New generation antidepressants such as mianserin or dothiepen are better tolerated since they produce fewer side-effects than the more established tricyclic antidepressants, such as amitriptyline. This is an important consideration for patients who may already be experiencing untoward effects from their disease and/or its treatment. Patients should be warned that antidepressants do not work immediately, and that a mood-elevating effect may not be noticed for up to two weeks. It is important to ensure that an adequate dose is maintained for as long as possible, ideally several months, to minimize the risk of relapse of depression. Patients should be warned of side-effects, especially drowsiness, and told that they are not simply receiving a tranquillizer.

2 *Psychological support*
Many patients need to talk through problems which may

otherwise tend to maintain their depression. For instance, feelings about disease progression or fears about terminal illness may need to be ventilated and the patient helped to cope. It may be necessary to facilitate 'unfinished business' between a patient and her partner, or counsel relatives about the patient's problems. For instance, a patient may wish to discuss future provision for her children, or even give her spouse 'permission' to remarry after her death, but finds her husband blocks any attempt to talk about these painful topics. Here, the partner may be using avoidance as a means of coping and will need considerable support and understanding himself in working through these issues.

Some women will require a more intensive approach using cognitive therapy in which they are taught problem-solving strategies and a technique to identify and overcome their negative thoughts. This can help re-establish a sense of self-mastery in a situation in which the patient often feels out of control.

Anxiety states **1** *Anxiolytic medication*
The benzodiazepines, though now unpopular with some patients, remain an effective group of drugs for the relief of anxiety. When prescribed for short courses and discontinued under supervision, dependence can be avoided. They have also proved of value in the premedication and sedation of patients receiving parenteral chemotherapy, and may help to alleviate conditioned nausea and vomiting by controlling the underlying anxiety.

When benzodiazepines are unsuitable, or if agitation occurs associated with depression, a major tranquillizer such as chlorpromazine is appropriate. Patients should be warned of possible extrapyramidal side-effects with these drugs.

In patients in whom somatic symptoms of anxiety predominate a betablocker such as propranolol may be the drug of choice.

2 *Behavioural treatment*
An increasing number of patients wish to learn to control anxiety symptoms, rather than rely on medication, and for them relaxation training is an effective strategy. Progressive muscular relaxation is one of several approaches to relaxation; for its success patients must be motivated to practise the techniques, and audiotaped instructions are helpful.

Relaxation is also a basis for the behavioural management of conditioned vomiting, in which 'desensitization' to the feared situation may also be used.

Organic brain syndrome The priority in management is to establish the underlying cause and correct it whenever the problem is reversible. In the meantime, agitated patients often require sedation, and for this a major tranquillizer such as haloperidol or chlorpromazine should be used. A single agent is preferable to a drug combination; starting with a small dose initially, it should be administered frequently (every hour or two if necessary) and the dose titrated against the patient's behaviour. Thereafter, a steady 4–6 hourly dose regimen may be established. Patients should be quietly nursed in a well-lit room, and frequently reminded of the correct orientation to help them return to normality.

Controversies and Future Developments
- The easy identification of patients with psychological morbidity.
- Evaluation of interventional therapies.
- The widespread introduction of counselling support.

Further reading

Altmaier, E.M., Ross, W.E. & Moore, K. (1982) A pilot investigation of the psychologic functioning of patients with anticipatory vomiting. *Cancer, 49*, 201–204.

Baum, M., Priestman, T., West, R. & Jones, E. (1980) A comparison of subjective responses in a trial comparing endocrine with cytotoxic treatment in advanced carcinoma of the breast. *Eur. J. Cancer, Suppl. 1*, 223–226.

DeHaes, J.C.J.M., Pruyn, J.F.A. & Van Knippenberg, F.C.E. (1983) Klachtenlijst voor kankerpatienten. Eerste ervaringen. *Nederlands Tijdschrift voor de Psychologie, 38*, 403–422.

Farber, J.M., Weinerman, B.H. & Kuypers, J.A. (1982) Psychological adjustment in oncology out patients. *Proc. Am. Soc. Clin. Oncol., 1*, 45, Abstract c-177.

Goldberg, D.P. (1972) *The Detection of Psychiatric Illness by Questionnaire.* London: Oxford University Press.

Hinton, J. (1972) Psychiatric consultation in fatal illness. *Proc. R. Soc. Med., 65*, 1035–1040.

Levine, P.M., Silberfarb, P.M. & Lipowski, Z.J. (1978) Mental disorders in cancer patients. *Cancer, 42*, 1385–1391.

Maguire, G.P., Tait, A., Brooke, M., Thomas, C. & Sellwood, R. (1980) Effect of counselling on the psychiatric morbidity associated with mastectomy. *Br. Med. J., 281*, 1454–1456.

Massie, M.S., Gorzynski, G., Mastrovito, G., Holland, J. & Theis, D. (1979) The diagnosis of depression in hospitalized patients with cancer. *Proc. Am. Ass. Cancer Res.* and *Am. Soc. Clin. Oncol., 20*, 432, Abstract c-587.

Nesse, R.M., Cark, T., Curtis, G.C. & Kleinman, P.D. (1980) Pretreatment nausea in cancer chemotherapy; a conditioned response? *Psychosom. Med., 42*, 33–36.

Plumb, M.M. & Holland, J. (1981) Comparative studies of psychological function in patients with advanced cancer. II. Interviewer-rated current and past psychiatric symptoms. *Psychosom. Med., 43*, 243–254.

Zigmond, A.S. & Snaith, R.P. (1983) The hospital anxiety and depression scale. *Acta Psychiat. Scand., 67*, 361–370.

31 Introduction to Benign Breast Disease

Roger Blamey

There is no strict definition of benign breast disease: on the one hand there is a symptom (breast pain) with no pathological correlate, on the other hand there are breast lumps which would not give rise to any anxiety if it were not for the presentation of breast cancer as a lump. The formation of cysts and the assumption of the fibrocystic histological changes of mammary dysplasia (Fig. 31.1), can be regarded as normal in women from the age of around 35–50. Younger women probably form fibroadenomata in very many cases, the majority remaining impalpable.

In the following chapters three complications of benign breast disease are separately discussed: fibroadenoma (this presents as a lump and conventionally, therefore, requires operative excision), breast pain and the woman who is plagued by multiple cyst formation. These are the three chief complications of benign breast disease that require treatment.

The other management complications are the presentation of an apparent lump, which on histology proves to show only fibrocystic change; entities which present through mammography with suspicion of cancerous change (Chapters 3 and 8); and histological changes which are precancerous (cellular atypia).

Figure 31.1
Low power view of cystic mammary dysplasia. H&E×126.

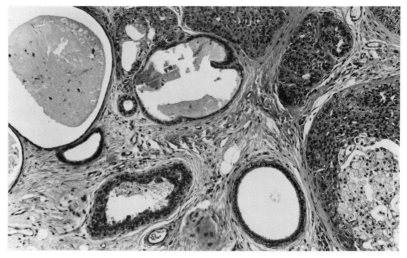

This latter subject has been a topic of debate for many years and is discussed in Chapter 2.

If I should seem to have been somewhat dismissive of benign breast disease in this short introductory chapter, it is worth remembering that in our breast clinic some 1800 patients will be referred each year with what proves to be benign breast disease. Most require reassurance, but many require investigation (including surgical biopsy in around 150 cases) before it may be given. Some present for treatment of breast pain (Chapter 32) or of duct ectasia with recurrent infection (Chapter 4): around 50 per annum will be treated for these conditions.

Benign breast disease, however defined, is a common complaint and takes up a good deal of medical time for its management.

32 Breast Pain

Christopher Hinton

Pain in the breast is a common symptom. At some time in their reproductive life most women suffer from varying degrees of premenstrual breast pain and tenderness. For some the appearance of such symptoms or a change in the severity or character of the pain causes anxiety as it is taken to be a manifestation of breast cancer. In others the severity of the pain itself presents unacceptable strictures to their life.

The significance of the complaint of breast pain as a presenting symptom in a breast clinic can be gauged from a survey which has been performed of 1500 patients referred as new cases to the Nottingham City Hospital Breast Clinic in 1979. During this year 25% of all patients presented with breast pain either in isolation or in association with other breast symptoms.

The classification of breast pain
The correct management of patients with breast pain relies on the accurate classification of patients into groups from which treatment follows logically. In many cases the precise mechanism by which the pain is caused is not well understood and the classification therefore must in part be empirical, being based on the results of treatment. Nevertheless, accurate classification is possible and greatly simplifies the management of patients and improves the therapeutic results. The first real attempt to classify breast pain was made by Preece et al (1976) who demonstrated that there were distinct patterns to breast pain. Subsequently, from Nottingham we reported an attempt to use this classification in a prospective practical manner. The classification presented here is based on these reports. The causes of breast pain may be divided into three groups: (1) True breast pain; (2) Referred musculoskeletal pain; and (3) Miscellaneous other causes.

It must be stressed that this classification of pain applies only to women complaining of breast pain in the absence of other detectable abnormalities. Careful examination of the breast is mandatory in every case. Patients with lumps, nipple retraction or discharge, or skin dimpling which may be indicative of an underlying carcinoma, must be appropriately investigated.

True breast pain There are three distinct clinical entities which come under the heading of true breast pain: (1) cyclical breast pain, (2) continuous breast pain, (3) trigger spots.

1 *Cyclical breast pain*

This syndrome is by far the most common cause of breast pain seen in a breast clinic. It is characterized by pain which varies in intensity through the menstrual cycle, being particularly severe in the weeks leading up to menstruation and decreasing after the onset of menstruation. At its worst it may become continuous with only a decrease in intensity during the time of menstruation. Even in women who have had a hysterectomy these cyclical variations can be elicited (a diary in which pain is recorded on a day-to-day basis is helpful in this regard). With this consistent cyclical variation the syndrome must have an hormonal basis but the nature of the interaction between cyclical hormone changes and the breasts is unknown. Examination of these women usually reveals tender, nodular breasts. On occasions these nodular, lumpy breasts may cause diagnostic difficulty and it is often useful to re-examine the woman in the week following her next period when the nodularity is least prominent.

2 *Continuous breast pain*

This small group of women complain of pain in one or both breasts which does not and has never shown any cyclical variation in intensity. It is a diagnosis of exclusion made when other causes, such as pain referred from musculoskeletal origin, have been excluded. Examination of the breasts is usually unrewarding, although in a few the pain is associated with duct ectasia and the palpable ectatic ducts may be felt as a cord beneath the nipple.

3 *Trigger spot*

Some women presenting with breast pain complain of pain referred always to the same part of the breast which on examination is exquisitely tender. If the tender area can consistently be located to the same spot on repeated visits to the clinic, then these women can be empirically treated by excision of the tender area. Histological examination of the excised portion of breast tissue frequently shows the changes of benign mammary dysplasia but no more specific cause for the pain is ever found.

Musculo-skeletal pain

1 *Cervical root syndrome*

Root pain from the lower cervical or upper thoracic spine can be associated with the complaint of pain in the breast. In most patients the diagnosis is not difficult once it has been considered since the pain also extends into the neck over the shoulder and down the arm and is not infrequently associated with paraesthesia. Investigations include cervical spine and thoracic inlet X-rays, which may show evidence of degenerative disease or an unexpected cervical rib.

2 *Tietze's syndrome (costochondritis)*
Tietze in 1921 first documented the condition of painful swelling of the costochondral cartilages, which in some cases was mistaken for breast carcinoma. More commonly, swelling is not a prominent feature and patients complain of pain only. These patients frequently present to the breast clinic, but the diagnosis can be made by eliciting tenderness over the affected costochondral junctions and not in the breast tissue itself.

Miscellaneous This group of patients includes a wide variety of pathological conditions. Patients with angina, biliary colic and reflux oesophagitis have all presented to the breast pain clinic. Two groups of patients within this classification are worthy of particular consideration.

Breast pain may be one of the first symptoms of pregnancy. Once the diagnosis is considered it is easy to make. There is often a characteristic feel to the breasts in early pregnancy and palpation may suggest the appropriate investigation.

Patients with breast pain have often been described as neurotic and the symptoms taken to be a sign of psychological rather than physical disturbance. Preece, however, has been able to show that they are no more neurotic than matched women presenting to a varicose veins clinic (Preece et al, 1978) and it is to do no service to the majority of women with breast pain to dismiss them as such. Nevertheless, there are a small number of women with psychological or psychosexual disorders who present to the breast pain clinic for whom physical treatment would be inappropriate despite their strenuous demands and who should, if they can be persuaded, be referred for psychiatric assessment.

The treatment of breast pain
Most patients with breast pain require no specific treatment. With the majority of women presenting with breast pain to the breast clinic simple reassurance, coupled with advice on good support (a maternity bra or sports bra is appropriate) which should be worn day and night during the painful part of the menstrual cycle, together with advice on simple analgesia, is sufficient to relieve their anxiety and control their pain. Many patients presenting to General Practitioners with mild breast pain are prescribed an oral contraceptive or diuretic. Neither have been shown to be effective. (Indeed some patients experience an exacerbation of symptoms with oral contraceptives.) At best, a placebo response may be obtained and side-effects may be encountered. Neither contraceptive nor diuretic is a substitute for careful examination and the reassurance this can provide. If the simple measures described above fail to adequately control symptoms, then and only then should women be referred for treatment.

In approximately 10% of patients referred with breast pain, the discomfort is sufficiently severe to interfere with their life and to warrant treatment in its own right. In these patients the first step to successful management is correct classification.

Referred musculo-skeletal pain

1 *Cervical root syndrome*
If simple analgesia fails to control the pain a regime of physiotherapy to the neck and shoulder girdle is prescribed, followed by a cervical collar to be worn at night if necessary.

2 *Tietze's syndrome*
Time is the great healer in these patients and once again simple analgesia is often all that is required. In patients with severe pain which is resistant to treatment with simple analgesia, injection of the affected costochondral joint with lignocaine and Depo-Medrone (2 ml of a mixture of lignocaine 1% and Depo-Medrone 40 mg) has proved effective.

True breast pain

1 *Trigger spots*
True trigger spots are uncommon. They are most often a localized manifestation of generalized breast disease in that the pain is cyclical in origin and should be treated as such. In those patients in whom there is consistent localized tenderness sufficient to be deemed a trigger spot, local excision of the painful area is the treatment of choice. Before embarking on this procedure, the patient should be seen on several occasions in the clinic to confirm that the location of the painful area is consistent over a period of months. Preoperatively, some time needs to be spent in careful marking of the area to be excised by the surgeon who is to perform the procedure and the patient must realize that despite this there is no guarantee of success. Even in the most expert hands, and with careful patient selection, up to 20% of these patients will have further trouble following excision.

2 *Continuous breast pain*
Patients complaining of continuous breast pain are frequently difficult to manage. Some are responsive to treatments applicable to cyclical breast pain and a therapeutic trial of these agents may be useful. In a few the condition is associated with palpable ectatic ducts, with or without nipple discharge. In some there is marked tenderness of the palpable ducts or evidence of infection, and antibiotics may be of value. In the absence of such signs, patients may be offered surgical excision of the major duct system if the pain is confined to the nipple area. In the majority of patients, however, analgesia is all that can be offered short of mastectomy.

3 *Cyclical breast pain*
Of patients presenting with true breast pain by far the largest

number have cyclical breast pain. Much attention has been focused on the management of this condition. Two agents in particular have been suggested as being effective in cyclical breast pain. These are the antigonadotrophin, danazol, and the antiprolactin agent, bromocriptine. Experience in a double-blind controlled trial performed in the Nottingham breast pain clinic has resulted in the choice of danazol as the first-line treatment for patients with severe cyclical breast pain which is resistant to simple measures. The regimen used begins with 300 mg danazol daily, the dose being gradually reduced over three months to 100 mg daily. In most patients a three month course has been sufficient but a few require maintenance treatment and for these purposes 100 mg danazol per day in the second half of the menstrual cycle is usually sufficient to produce long-term control. We now restrict the use of bromo-criptine to those patients in whom there is a contraindication to danazol therapy (obesity or migraine), in whom there are side-effects while taking danazol (headaches, weight gain or muscle cramps), or in whom danazol treatment has failed. Bromocriptine is started at a dose of 0.125 mg daily and this is gradually increased over a two week period to 0.25 mg given twice a day. In patients who fail to respond to one agent, treatment with other drugs is often disappointing, but a number of other agents may sometimes be helpful. These include tamoxifen (10 mg b.d.), norethisterone (5 mg t.d.s. in the second half of the menstrual cycle) and Efamol (evening primrose oil, 6 capsules daily).

The role of mastectomy in the management of breast pain

Consideration of the management of breast pain would not be complete without giving some thought to the role of mastectomy. Many patients with intractable breast pain which is resistant to treatment ultimately suggest mastectomy as a possible answer. The vast majority of patients, even with the severest breast pain, can be adequately managed by drug treatment or minor surgical procedures and all of these means should be first exhausted. Before considering subcutaneous or simple mastectomy, the clinician must be convinced that there is a physical cause for the pain which is within the breast and cannot be managed by other means. All patients should have appropriate investigations including cervical spine X-ray, thoracic inlet X-ray and mammography, and all possible causes of referred pain must be sought. In the Nottingham breast pain clinic this psychiatric assessment is a precondition of consideration for mastectomy. Once these conditions have been fulfilled, subcutaneous or simple mastectomy may be successful, but in our experience some patients have continued to complain of the same symptoms as they experienced preoperatively and for this reason mastectomy is offered only as a last resort and with great reluctance.

Problems in the management of breast pain

Pain as a symptom of primary breast carcinoma

Much has been written of the importance of breast pain as a symptom of breast carcinoma, and a number of patients with a primary breast cancer do experience pain in the breast. In the survey of patients presenting to the Nottingham City Hospital Breast Clinic in 1979, 48 of the 192 patients with breast cancer complained of associated breast pain. In all but one of these patients careful clinical examination revealed other associated abnormalities suggestive of breast cancer; in only 1 of 446 patients presenting with breast pain was this the only presenting feature of breast cancer.

The side-effects of drug treatments

Many of the treatments of cyclical breast pain involve hormonal manipulation and it is not therefore surprising that many have associated side-effects. Most side-effects are of a minor nature and problems can be avoided by careful discussion with the patient before commencing treatment.

Danazol

The antigonadotrophin danazol appears to have a multifactoral mode of action. Its principal effect is to block the synthesis and storage of gonadotrophins. It suppresses the normal hormone cycle and in sufficient doses will produce amenorrhoea.

In the dosage normally used in the treatment of breast pain, the effect on menstruation is inconsistent. In the majority, normal menstruation proceeds throughout treatment. In some women amenorrhoea results from doses as low as 100 mg/day but more commonly menstrual irregularity is produced. If patients are warned that this may occur, it seldom causes more than minor inconvenience and never requires withdrawal of treatment.

Danazol has a mild androgenic activity which may play a part in its efficacy in the treatment of cyclical breast pain. Probably as a result of this activity, there is a tendency for patients treated with danazol to gain weight. The tendency is dose-related. In most the weight gain is modest and easily lost when treatment stops, but the patient should be warned of this possibility and weight should be monitored during treatment, particularly in obese patients.

In patients with true migraine, danazol often produces an increase in the frequency of attacks and a history of classic migraine is a contraindication to therapy.

Other side-effects are uncommon at the dosage level used in the management of cyclical breast pain. Occasionally, patients complain of muscle cramps which necessitate withdrawal of the drug and in long-term use at high dosages reversible changes in complexion and hirsutism may be seen.

Bromocriptine

Side-effects associated with the use of bromocriptine are considerably reduced by increasing the dose gradually at the start of treatment. All are dose-dependent and decrease after a period of time. Most common are headaches, dizziness, nausea and vomiting, and constipation. If patients are warned and told to expect these symptoms to improve with time, treatment seldom needs to be withdrawn. It is usually sufficient to delay any increment in dosage. One particularly distressing side-effect is sometimes seen. That is, postural hypotension which may result in sudden collapse. To minimize the possibility of this occurrence, treatment is initiated as a small dose taken at night so that the maximal effect is achieved during sleep and only later is the dosage increased and a daytime dose introduced. While an episode of postural hypotension is not necessarily an indication for withdrawal of treatment, patients are seldom willing to try again.

Other drugs
Side-effects are uncommon with the other drugs used in the management of cyclical breast pain, but the possibility of the cystic ovarian changes occasionally reported with high doses of tamoxifen suggest that this drug should be used with caution.

Contraceptive advice

Of the above drugs only Efamol can be considered suitable in pregnancy. Pregnancy should be excluded prior to other treatments and patients advised to take contraceptive precautions. Since hormonal contraceptives are likely to interact with these therapeutic agents, contraception should be by a barrier method or intrauterine device.

Risk of subsequent breast cancer

Many histological features of benign breast disease have been suggested as indicators of the risk of the subsequent development of breast cancer. There is no evidence of an association between breast pain (of whatever nature) and any particular histological features. At this time, therefore, breast pain cannot be considered to be an indication of any increase in the risk of subsequent breast cancer.

Summary
Patients with mild breast pain can be managed by conservative means. Rarely is it the sole presenting symptom in breast cancer. In those with more persistent or severe pain, management is simplified by accurate classification such that the appropriate treatment suggests itself.

The largest group are those with cyclical breast pain. The aetiology of cyclical breast pain is unclear but must be of an hormonal nature. In patients with cyclical breast pain resistant to conservative treatment, the antigonadotrophin danazol is the treatment of choice. Side-effects of treatment are not uncommon but usually do not necessitate withdrawal of treatment.

There is no evidence that breast pain is an indicator of increased risk of subsequent breast cancer.

Further reading

Bishop, H.M. & Blamey, R.W. (1979) A suggested classification of breast pain. *Postgrad. Med. J.*, *55 (5)*, 59–60.

Preece, P.E., Mansel, R.E., Bolton, P.M. et al (1976) Clinical syndromes of mastalgia. *Lancet*, *ii*, 670.

Preece, P.E., Mansel, R.E. & Hughes, L.E. (1978) Mastalgia: psychoneurosis or organic disease? *Br. Med. J.*, *1*, 29–30.

33 Fibroadenoma

Paul Preece

Many of the operations carried out for benign breast disease involve the removal of fibroadenomas, most commonly from young women. Inevitably a proportion of these develop painful postoperative haematomas, wound infections and unsightly scars. An average district general hospital will perform 50 such operations per year, at the cost to the patients of these sequelae. Do fibroadenomas really need to be removed?

The overwhelming reason that benign conditions of the breast are of importance is the possible existence of malignant disease. Any abnormality observed or suspected in a breast gives rise to three concerns: (1) Is the cause malignancy? (2) Will any lesion present become malignant? (3) Is there an increased predisposition to malignancy?

Clinical features

Fibroadenomas present clinically as lumps palpable in the developed breast. They are characteristically definite to feel, that is they are discrete, hard, smooth, usually spherical, and mobile. This last feature has caused them to be nicknamed 'breast mice'. It is not unusual for them to be multiple. Most commonly, they develop during young adulthood, that is from between puberty and 25 years of age. This observation is the single most important consideration in avoiding misdiagnosis.

Although fibroadenomas are detected clinically and mammographically in the breasts of older women, these probably arose during their young adulthood. It is easy to understand that pre-existing lesions could become palpable within breasts which are involuting with age. Fibroadenomas are usually slow growing. The majority which are clinically detectable stop growing once they have reached 1–3 cm in diameter. Thereafter, unless they are removed, they persist. A small proportion of fibroadenomas left in the breast continue to grow and become 'giants'. There is no clinical or cytological feature of these which enables them to be identified while they are still small. At least one in five patients who develop a fibroadenoma develop others either concurrently or successively.

Histology

Happily, there is no dispute about the tissue from which fibroadenomata are believed to originate. Although they contain an epithelial component, they are regarded as arising from

Figure 33.1
Photomicrograph of
pericanalicular
fibroadenoma.

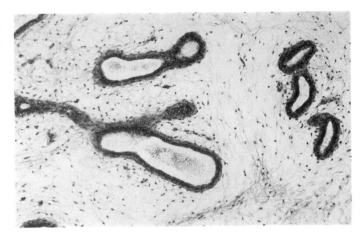

connective tissue. This does not preclude the possibility that it is the growth of the accompanying epithelium which is the factor controlling their growth. At puberty, the stroma of the breast grows. Fibroadenomas are localized foci of excess growth of connective tissue. The resulting appearances are so close morphologically to those of the normal stroma as to leave little doubt as to their origin.

The detailed classification made by Cutler (1961) explains the different microscopic appearances of these lumps. In summary, two appearances are distinguished: (1) pericanalicular and periacinous (Fig. 33.1), which are the commonest, usually seen between puberty and 25 years of age; and (2) subepithelial, which appear clinically between 30 and 50 years (Fig. 33.2).

Since fibroadenomas arise from connective tissue, it is not to be expected that they would become carcinomatous. Generally, this

Figure 33.2
Photomicrograph of
subepithelial
fibroadenoma.

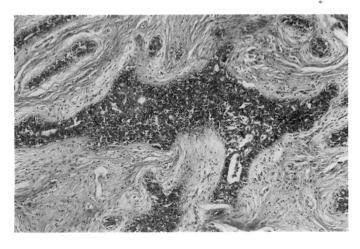

Figure 33.3
A typically cellular smear obtained by fine-needle aspiration from a fibroadenoma.

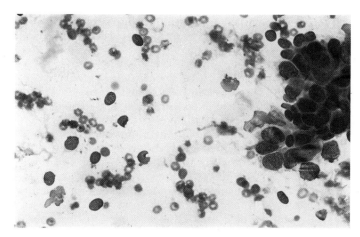

expectation is realized in practice and is supported by the literature. Clinical experience also confirms that sarcomatous change is extremely rare.

Cytology

Despite the relative simplicity of their histopathology, the cytology of fine-needle aspirates from fibroadenomas is not uniformly simple. In their favour, and perhaps surprisingly considering they are predominantly connective tissue neoplasms, they yield cellular smears. This means it is relatively easy to obtain technically satisfactory smears from them (Fig. 33.3). Less favourably, this very cellularity can itself cause difficulty in diagnosis, the cells on occasion having some characteristics of malignancy (Fig. 33.4). Both fibroadenomas and benign 'lumpiness' yield identical cellular elements on fine-

Figure 33.4
A smear from a fibroadenoma which has features mimicking malignancy (ultimate histology of lump confirmed as fibroadenoma).

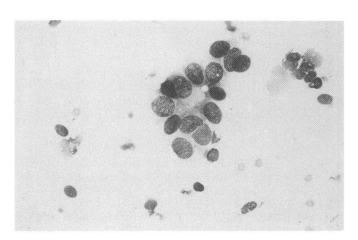

needle aspiration, but fibroadenomas are distinctive in that it is only these which yield naked bipolar nuclei.

Treatment
Unfortunately, the clinically clearcut entity, fibroadenoma, may be mimicked by breast cancer. The standard treatment is therefore excision. Some 800 fibroadenomas have been removed in Nottingham over the past 12 years; coincidentally no cancer in patients aged under 25 has been diagnosed but cancer occurred in 15 patients aged under 30 years. Several of these cancers were noted at the initial clinic examination as 'clear fibroadenomas'.

The fact that these operations are often regarded as minor and left in the hands of the least skilled member of the surgical team, increases the likelihood of haematoma and unsightly scars. General anaesthesia is preferable, since local anaesthetic may give difficulty in the location of small lumps. Breast tissue in young women is always vascular and coagulation diathermy, usually used plentifully, is the best and often the only way to obtain adequate haemostasis; the bleeding from the cut breast is frequently a generalized ooze, rather than seepage from an identifiable vessel.

Excision should be through a small circumferential (i.e. skin crease) incision, placed if possible on the margin of the areola. The lump can be stabilized either by inserting into it a hypodermic needle before the incision is made, or by transfixing it with a heavy needle mounted ligature after the skin has been incised. The latter enables traction to be applied to the lump without its being fragmented by tissue forceps, and further facilitates haemostasis which can be achieved by diathermy with complete control as dissection proceeds. Where this has not been achieved, then a small suction drain should be placed from the resulting cavity. A drain will normally necessitate an overnight stay in hospital but this might be avoided if the procedure can be performed as a day case. A good cosmetic result can be achieved by closing the skin with a fine (e.g. 3/0 or 4/0) monofilament polypropylene subcuticular suture, which should be removed after six or seven days, or by using the same material as interrupted sutures, replaced on the fourth postoperative day with small self-adhesive paper skin closures.

The real question is: 'Can we avoid excision of these benign lesions altogther?' It is probably safe to do so provided the following criteria are strictly observed:

1 The patient is under 25 years of age.

2 The clinical characteristics of the lump are as described above, and the patient herself has not been aware of any increase in its size.

3 Fine-needle aspiration is always performed and the cells seen are unequivocally normal.

Summary

A policy of leaving fibroadenomas unoperated is currently being tested in Dundee and Nottingham, using cytological as well as clinical criteria to make this diagnosis. At present those discrete 'fibroadenoma-like lumps' that should be removed are:

- those developing newly at age 25 years or over
- those which have grown rapidly
- those which are at presentation very large (i.e. > 3 cm)
- those with very cellular stroma on cytology
- those giving abnormal epithelial cytology
- those which the patient wishes removed despite assurance from the surgeon

In the future, as experience and confidence with cytology increases, it is possible that, using two or three separate fine-needle aspirations, the age limit for leaving these lesions will be expanded upwards and the majority of fibroadenomas will be left in situ. At present this is not recommended.

Controversies and Future Developments
- Using a combination of fine-needle aspiration cytology (but note the expertise required – Chapter 1), careful clinical assessment and follow-up, mammography and possibly a further physical investigation (eg. lite-scan), it should prove possible to make the excision of benign lumps unnecessary.

Further reading

Cutler, M. (1961) *Fibroadenoma Tumours of the Breast*, pp. 384–408. Philadelphia: J.B. Lipincott.

Schöndorf, H. (1978) *Aspiration Cytology of the Breast*, p. 70. Philadelphia: W.B. Saunders.

34 Recurrent Breast Cysts

Christopher Hinton

In premenopausal women over the age of 30 years, cysts are the most common cause of breast lumps in women presenting to a breast clinic. Most can be successfully dealt with by simple aspiration. Aspiration serves not only to exclude the diagnosis of carcinoma but in most cases it produces permanent resolution of the breast cyst. Providing that the palpable mass disappears after aspiration of the cyst and the cyst fluid is not blood stained, no further action is necessary if the cyst does not recur. In some patients, however, repeated recurrence of a single cyst, or the appearance of multiple cysts throughout both breasts, presents a management problem.

According to the criteria laid down by Patey and still largely adhered to, repeated recurrence of a single breast cyst is an indication for excision to exclude the possibility of an intracystic carcinoma. It is the natural history of some cysts to recur and very few will contain any form of intracystic lesion. It is in the interests of both the patient and the surgical work load to avoid excision if such a lesion can be excluded.

Approximately 10% of all patients with breast cysts make repeated visits to the clinic with multiple cysts at different sites in one or both breasts. In these women the repeated finding of a lump in the breast causes considerable anxiety and the repeated aspiration of these cysts is time-consuming for the clinician and unpleasant for the patient.

The management of recurrent breast cysts

The single recurrent breast cyst
If a residual lump is present following aspiration of a breast cyst then this must be excised. This principle applies however many times that the cyst has been drained.

It has been conventional to excise cysts which recur or in which the aspirate is blood-stained in order to exclude the presence of an intracystic lesion. Intracystic carcinoma is rare and blood-staining of the fluid is more often due to needle trauma during aspiration. Recurrence is most commonly from a simple cyst recurrence or the appearance of a second cyst in an anatomically indistinguishable site.

Three forms of investigation may be helpful:

1 *The pneumocystogram*
Routine mammography following cyst aspiration is generally unhelpful and may be misleading if there is oedema at the

aspiration site. In a patient with a recurrent breast cyst a pneumocystogram is simple to perform and can be used to exclude intracystic pathology (see Chapter 8). Following cyst aspiration, without withdrawing the needle, a quantity of air equal to the amount of fluid aspirated is instilled into the cyst. The patient is then sent for two view mammography of the breast. The cyst can be seen in negative outline and the internal lining of the cyst visualized.

2 *Ultrasound*
Ultrasound examination of the breast (which must be performed prior to cyst aspiration) may also be helpful in detecting intracystic lesions. Breast ultrasound must be performed by an experienced operator on an appropriate ultrasound scanner.

3 *Cytological examination of the cyst fluid*
This has not proved helpful in several large series.

The criteria for operation on a cyst put forward above now appears out of date. Residual lumps and uniformly bloody taps must be subjected to excision biopsy but, provided investigation provides no evidence of intracystic pathology, the remainder of these recurrent cysts can be safely subjected to repeated aspiration.

Multiple recurrent breast cysts

A few patients with breast cysts make repeated visits to the breast clinic with multiple cysts occurring throughout the breasts. Although these patients can be managed by repeated aspiration this is time-consuming and unpleasant and there would be a case for treating some of these women if an effective treatment was available.

There is an obvious hormonal association in the aetiology of breast cysts as evidenced by the virtual disappearance of breast cysts following the menopause. This has led to the investigation of the use of the antigonoadotrophin, danazol, in the management of these women with multiple recurrent breast cysts.

Table 34.1
The results of a trial investigating the use of danazol in patients with multiple recurrent breast cysts.

	Total	No. forming cysts	No. with no cyst formation
Controls	15	13	2
Danazol-treated	18	6*	12

$P < 0.0001$ on chi-squared test.
* Including two patients who did not receive a full course of treatment.

Figure 34.1
Mammographic
appearance of breast
of patient before (a)
and after (b) three
months of danazol
treatment.

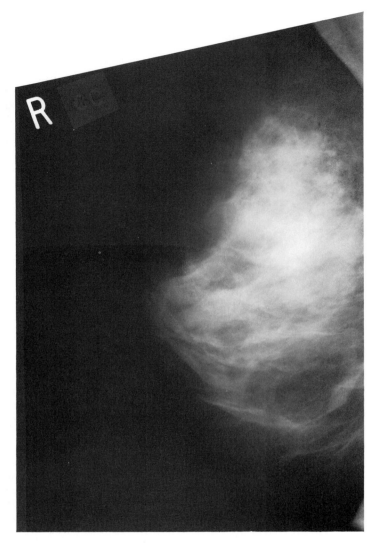

a

In a controlled trial at the Nottingham City Hospital Breast Clinic, patients with multiple recurrent breast cysts were randomized to receive either no treatment or danazol, 100 mg t.d.s., for three months. All patients had had multiple breast cysts which had required repeated aspiration over a period greater than six months. On entry into the trial, palpable cysts were drained and mammography performed (Fig. 34.1) so that the number of residual cysts in the breast could be counted. Patients were seen at three months and palpable cysts were drained. All patients were then seen again in a further three months. Palpable cysts were once again drained and further mammography performed. The number of cysts which had formed over the six month period

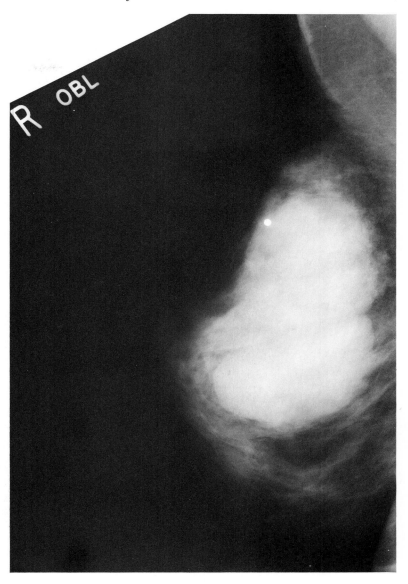

b

was calculated by adding the total number of cysts aspirated to the number seen on the final mammogram and subtracting from this the number of residual cysts which had been seen at their initial attendance on mammography. Of the patients allocated to the control group, 13 out of 15 formed cysts during the period of study: only 4 out of 18 of the danazol group formed cysts (Table 34.1). Most of the remainder in this group had net resolution of cysts over the period of study. This net resolution was not only accounted for by a resolution of the mammographically detected impalpable cysts. The patients in the treated group not only required less frequent cyst aspiration but also had fewer cysts aspirated on each occasion. Although danazol is known to have some side-effects, none of these patients suffered untoward effects necessitating withdrawal of the drug.

Further work is required to define the role of danazol in the management of these women, particularly regarding the optimum length of treatment and the need for maintenance therapy, but from the results available danazol appears to be effective, at least in the short term, and may be valuable in the treatment of women with multiple recurrent breast cysts.

Aetiology

The cysts with a high sodium:potassium ratio and a low DHA sulphate concentration have a lining consisting of basophilic cells with little cytoplasm which has been termed a 'flattened epithelium': cysts with a low sodium : potassium ratio and a high DHA sulphate concentration have a lining of acidophilic cells with copious granular cytoplasm which has been termed 'apocrine epithelium' (Dixon et al, 1983). It is from the latter group that the recurrent cyst-formers come. Aprocrine change in breast epithelium in the ducts and lobules has been suggested as being a major risk factor (Wellings et al, 1975) for the subsequent development of carcinoma but further work is required to confirm this.

Summary

Two distinct problems arise in the management of patients with breast cysts: the solitary recurrent cyst in which there may be a suspicion of an intracystic lesion, and multiple recurrent cysts causing patients anxiety and requiring repeated out-patient consultations.

Where a residual lump is present after aspiration, excision biopsy is mandatory. For the remainder of patients with single recurrent cysts, careful examination and investigation using pneumocystography and/or ultrasound will in most cases render excision of the cyst unnecessary.

In patients presenting repeatedly with cysts at different sites in one or both breasts, treatment with the antigonadotrophin, danazol, has proved to be effective at least in the short term.

References

Dixon, J., Miller, W.R., Scott, W.N. & Forrest, A.P.M. (1983) The morphological basis of human breast cyst populations. *Br. J. Surg.*, 70, 604–606.

Hinton, C.P., Williams, M.R., Roebuck, E.J. & Blamey, R.W. (1986) A controlled trial of danazol in the treatment of multiple recurrent breast cysts. *Br. J. Clin. Pract.* (in press).

Wellings, S.R., Jensen, H.M. & Marcum, R.G. (1975). An atlas of subgross pathology of the human breast with reference to possible precancerous lesions. *J. Natl. Cancer Inst.*, 55, 231–275.

Index